T0036315

THE ART OF BINDING PEOPLE

Paolo Milone

THE ART OF BINDING PEOPLE

Translated from the Italian
by Lucy Rand

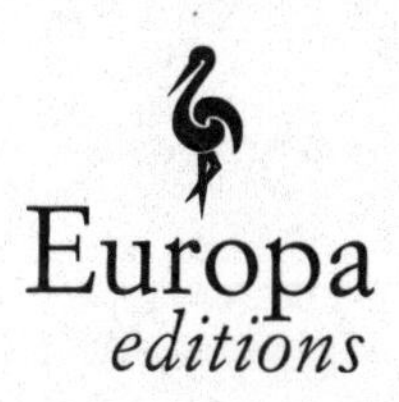

Europa Editions
27 Union Square West, Suite 302
New York NY 10003
www.europaeditions.com
info@europaeditions.com

First Publication 2023 by Europa Editions

Translation by Lucy Rand
Original title: *L'arte di legare le persone*

Library of Congress Cataloging in Publication Data is available
ISBN 978-1-60945-833-1

Milone, Paolo
The Art of Binding People

Art direction by Emanuele Ragnisco
instagram.com/emanueleragnisco

Cover design by Ginevra Rapisardi

Original artwork by Giulio Einaudi editore.
Adapted from Egon Schiele, *Self-portrait with Shirt*, Gouache 1910
Vienna, Leopold Museum (Photo © Akg Images / Mondadori Portfolio)

Prepress by Grafica Punto Print – Rome

Printed in Canada

CONTENTS

THE ART OF BINDING PEOPLE

1.

Having avoided every other job out of fear,
I find myself in the job everyone fears the most.

Chapter One
Ward 77

I.

I walk around the new psychiatric ward for the first time,
they've forgotten the interview rooms.
Like building a surgical ward without operating rooms.
Where are we to conduct interviews? I ask.
Dumbstruck they stare at me, what a question.
Interviews? In the patients' rooms, for God's sake.
I tell them that a surgeon, in the patient's room, changes dress-
ings, removes stitches and listens to the stomach,
but for operations he needs an operating room.
I, a psychiatrist, at the patient's bedside, say hello,
offer pleasantries, a friendly squeeze on the cheek,
play the fool, a big smile.
I may be young, but I know this much:
for interviews, I need an interview room, for God's sake.

2.

I insisted on having an interview room.
They responded that there was no budget for extravagances.
Extravagance? An interview room is an empty room.

3.

They take the brooms out of a broom cupboard and say to me,
Will this do for your interview room?
It's too small.
Use the dining room then.
It's too big.
What do you want?

An interview room must not be too big, nor too small.
It must not be too bright, nor too dark.
It must not be too noisy, nor too quiet.
It's too difficult, I realize. It's a magic room.
I'll never have an interview room.

4.

Yesterday a group of administrators came to see the new psychiatric ward and they liked it. How big the patients' rooms are! Then, euphoric and noisy, they set off for other shores.

And I thought, the euphoric are ambitious, impudent and tireless, euphoria gets you ahead.
But as soon as they reach a certain position they get bored and, rather than managing, they look around thinking, what am I doing here?
They're already thinking about where to go next.
This is their limit: they need to keep moving.
That's why administrators believe, in good faith and ignorance, that the patients love space. Space has, for them, an entirely positive value.
But it isn't true.

Euphoria is just one of many mental disorders:
in some of them the patient is indifferent to space,
in others, unthinkable but true, space distresses them.
The world is full of depressed people who sleep on sofas without even getting into pajamas,
or on the edge of the bed without pulling back the sheets, many sleep on chairs.
If you give them a double bed, it will remain untouched a month later.
They prefer it that way. It isn't external space they need.

5.

I walk into enormous empty rooms,
I see the patient in the bed in the distance,
across square feet of nothing
that are swollen with madness, where infinite worlds coexist,
and, after a long journey through silence,
I arrive at the island of desperation,
the master has already woken the dogs
and unsheathed his knife.
When I arrive I am tired and defenseless.
I don't know what to say or do.
I ought to retreat toward firm land,
and abandon this lifeboat in the infinite sea.

6.

Every morning is a thrill,
three bulletproof doors to go to work.
I imagine entering a nuclear power plant, fuel rods immersed in heavy water,

or the vaults of the Bank of Italy, bulging with gold and platinum bars,
or the cyclotron, a thousand yards beneath the Gran Sasso,
or Spectre's secret hiding place, full of white cats,
or the laboratories where they study Ebola.
Instead, disappointment.
After opening the first, the second, the third door,
I am greeted by the familiar faces of Giovanni, Lidia and Antonio.

7.

Talk of cutting the number of beds on the ward is met by a general sense of happiness.
The administrators are happy because they'll spend less,
the nurses are happy because they'll work less.
But I, a doctor, what do I have to be happy about?
Working less?

So I wander the empty spaces, listen to the rain falling, the trees being blown against the window.
It's the new Psychiatry. There is none. What joy.

8.

When I was a young psychiatrist at the Mental Health Center, people were amazed if I went into a room to talk with a patient.
They weren't used to that on psychiatric wards, they thought it an academic peculiarity.
Every time, just as I had started an interview, the door would creak open without warning

and someone would pop their head around, just curious.
Then a nurse would come in and pull out one, two, three drawers, rummage around for something he couldn't find and, without saying anything, leave again.
If I was with a woman, the head physician would appear personally to check we weren't having sex.
There was a constant coming and going: someone asking how long we needed the room for,
someone who had booked it for the afternoon, someone asking if they could use the telephone,
someone letting us know we'd been in there ten minutes.
Two people shutting themselves in a room to talk is strange. Disturbing.
Even in a Mental Health Center.

9.

On the new ward the ceilings have been adorned with smoke detectors and other electronic contraptions,
a spectacle of red, white and green lights flashing intermittently in the darkness of the night,
like on those magical country evenings when fireflies appear.

The third day after the opening, a paranoid person says to me—that's where they spy on us from.
In the patients' imaginations the little lights are video cameras, microphones, vents pumping poison into the air.
Yesterday I asked an administrator if the smoke detectors can't go somewhere else.
He looked at me like I was mad.

10.

I am about to go home when they bring you into the Emergency Room.
She's called Lucrezia, they tell me, she has cut her neck.
You greet me with the mocking smirk of a twenty-year-old.

Let me see your arms, I ask. You dodge.
I have to distract you with childish games to uncover your arms
and then, helped by two nurses, your underdeveloped body,
as you kick and spit, offended.
You have thirty fresh cuts from today, some deep.
Are you stupid? I shout in your face.
You stick out your tongue, then dig four nails into my flesh
and refuse to loosen your grip.

11.

To extract your nails from my arm,
I have to squeeze your hand hard and pull it away in the right direction.

I'm admitting you, I say. I don't want to. This is an involuntary hospitalization.
I just need to request permission at city hall and advise the guardianship judge—One hour and you're in the net, little fish.

My colleague from the ER appears at the door,
Hey, crazy people doctor,
admit this girl in psychiatry. I don't want lunatics walking around the ER!
I phone my ward and they tell me—There's no room!
Your diaphanous mother joins in—Admit her, I beg you!

Your drunk father joins in—I'm taking her home!
The on-call doctor reappears—Milone, get this girl off my ward!

I don't get ruffled, every day is like this.
I search only for your eyes, Lucrezia,
for a moment, they seem wiser than everyone else
then you join in—Uh-oh, psych, you're in trouble!

12.

Don't ask me, Anna, in the evening, why I look tired.
It is not because of the madness.
Madness is a garden where my tired horses drink, where I slip off my sandals, rest in the shade
and let my gaze fall on distant hills.
Don't ask me, in the evening, why my words are muddled.
It is not because of the madness.

13.

As soon as I enter Ward 77, dragging Lucrezia behind me, the nurse blocks my way—
Why are you admitting her if it's not what she wants?
It is what she wants.
But you're dragging her!
She has clawed me with her nails and won't let go,
it doesn't get plainer than that!
The nurse looks at me with big, incredulous eyes.

In Emergency Psychiatry, if you want to understand the patient, there has to be a physical struggle.

The person who understands the patient with whom I had the physical struggle,
is me, not you.

14.

Having just arrived on the ward,
Lucrezia barricades herself in the corridor, back to the wall
and begins to shout without letting up—I want to go home!
I whisper to the nurses—We need to restrain her, else she's going to hurt herself.
No, Massimo protests, a double injection, then she'll sleep.
We can't, I protest, she has low blood pressure, she might collapse.
O.K. so let's phone the head physician.

Why did you admit her? You shouldn't have brought her in!
I don't want involuntary hospitalizations on my ward!
I don't want anyone restrained on my ward!
If you can't use drugs, you'll have to stay with her all night until she falls asleep.

Lucrezia spends the night roaming the ward, shouting and keeping the world awake,
a nurse follows her around, sighing,
then at three the magic trick:
she pulls a blade out of nowhere and cuts her calves,
the only part of her body spared until now.

15.

If you have never experienced psychiatric pain,
do not say that it doesn't exist.

Thank the Lord and stop talking.

16.

Certain mornings, on Ward 77, you feel like you're on a Naples to Turin train in the 1950s.
Men and women squeezed between cardboard boxes, broken shoes, bottles of wine, a medley of smells and secretions,
a cigarette passed overhead, tissues, bread,
gazes lost in memories of the past or worries about the future.
A silent question, a nod, a touch, hair let down, a blow of the nose, sleeping, crying, staring into the void, thinking about fate with your face pressed into the glass.
The trees run in the wind. The train rattles.

What am I doing here?
I, passing between the mother with four children and the man with a three-day beard,
scratching at a wound with miner's hands,
I who know nothing.
Am I to be the conductor asking, tickets please?

17.

There are those who claim that a psychiatric admission is the worst thing in the world. But sometimes life is even worse.
When animals are wounded they hide in burrows and lick their wounds.
The psychiatric ward is the burrow.

18.

Ennio, at Christmas and at Easter you suffer from loneliness and admit yourself to Ward 77.
In among the mad people you feel at home, more than in your own home.
You stay for the holidays, then you leave.
Ennio, what happens to you at Christmas and Easter, happens to me every day.

19.

Emilio, you are like a child riding a bike downhill who doesn't know how to brake.
To stop, you have to crash into something: an angry husband, the police, a blocked credit card.
The people who love you are praying you'll crash sooner rather than later, that way you'll do yourself less harm.

When I met you, you had driven a car onto the beach
right up to the sea
and you were laughing at the fear on the faces of the bathers you nearly hit.
Your wife arrived at the Emergency Room, she burst into tears and repeated—At last! At last! Is the door to the ward locked with a key?
Yes.
Thank God.
Then came your daughter—At last! Is the door to the ward locked with a key?
Yes.
Thank God. At last.

Six months later you park your Porsche on the sidewalk, leave a blond at the bar,
run into my studio like a little boy.
You adjust the blue silk scarf around your neck.
Two imperfections: the scarf is conspicuously stained with grease and one arm of your glasses is held on with tape.

20.

Over time, we who work on Ward 77 become hardened to all sorts of strangeness.
To the stench of feet and urine, the broken tiles, broken doors, the screams, the cursing,
to the doctors and nurses who jostle around calling one another by their first names, to the patients bound to beds.
For the new patients arriving, however, it's always the first time.
So they look at us, wide-eyed with wonder, whatever we do.

21.

Filippo, you can't find the words to tell me what's happening to you and you look at me with anger, expectation, and remorse,
I, I can't find the words to explain what's happening to you,
and I can't find the words to calm you down.
Honestly, Filippo,
you're here, I'm here,
we're doing just fine.

22.

Lucrezia, the story you're trying to sell me about your suffering is a knockoff,
bought for a few pennies in the waiting room flea market
and you want to sell it on to me as if it's brand new!
I'm not falling for it. I won't buy.

23.

Lucrezia, you're still playing hide-and-seek with the razor blades.
I found one under a boob.
Another you were hiding in your pants.
The third in your mouth—too easy.
Game over, I win. Let's all go home, I'm already late.

Why do you have that crafty grin on your face? Show me your shoes!
I knew it: a four-pack.
The smile remains.
Hair. Let me feel your hair. Nothing. How many more do you have? Where are you hiding them?

I'll happily play hide-and-seek with cigarettes, lighters, alcohol, joints, even heroin and cocaine,
but I detest playing hide-and-seek with razor blades.
Lucrezia, you win, but tell me, where are they?

24.

When I was young it was stronger than me:

if I heard screaming on the ward I would have to run and check. The older nurses wouldn't move a muscle, but for me, trying to resist was useless. My legs would go on their own.
The nurses, silent, shot me disapproving looks.
I would leave the kitchen and do a round of the ward: everyone was fine.
Who's screaming, I'd ask. No response.
I'd go back to the nurses perplexed and they would pretend nothing had happened.
Another scream.
I'd try to stay still, but it was like a baby crying. My body would writhe in my seat.
Off to inspect the ward.
The fourth time I went, the nurses would speak with their eyes—
who knows if this boy will make it as a psychiatrist.

25.

Danilo, you're six-foot-seven tall and weight 240 pounds.
You're a young schizophrenic, but with an affectionate character.
The other day, you came into the room where I was writing a chart. I made the mistake of turning my back to you:
Milone, you know I like you right, really like you?
Two broken ribs.
Danilo, thank God you like me.

26.

At times I feel I'd like to be alone, one on one with madness, without this whirlwind of people clattering and clamoring around.

Dangerous desire.

27.

A Minotaur is roaming the Emergency Room.
He looks around nervously, sniffs the air, points his horns this way and that.
He exhales through his nostrils as he walks past the sacrificial altar.
His reddish-brown hair glimmers.
The smell of the forest rises upward.
From his broad chest comes a deep lament.

I, behind the curtain, have wrapped my head in a wreath of laurel,
washed my hands in pure water,
and dried them slowly.
And I step out.

28.

Psychiatry is screams and silent tears.

Once upon a time on the wards the patients screamed ceaselessly, for years on end. Now they scream on the first day, a little on the second, and on the third they are quiet.
Drugs—God bless them—have brought silence to the world.

But if we removed the drugs we'd be straight back there:
the heart of man would unleash screams and silent tears.

29.

When a farmer wants to show you something on his field, he extends his cane toward it and brushes it with the tip.
When, as a student, I shadowed an older psychiatrist for the first time in the Emergency Room,
he stopped at the doorway and examined the patient from four yards away.
There are two types of Psychiatry, long cane and short cane.

The vast world of Psychiatry opens up when you get to two yards from the patient.
If you get to one, it becomes phantasmagorical.
If you go any further, an inferno.

30.

If I see someone peeking over the edge,
I offer a hand so that they don't fall,
and as I hold them I ask what they see.
I am a coward:
I look into the abyss through the eyes of others.

31.

Giulia, come out of that room at once.
Two hours you've been alone with Lucrezia.
I realized too late: the milk is already boiling over the sides of the pan.
You are a young intern psychologist, you can't talk for two hours with a psychotic.

With her, for two hours, you can play cards, ball games, do some gardening, walk, watch TV, but not talk.
After an hour you'll be crazy.
Look at you, you look drugged.
Now go and wash your face, phone a friend and get some fresh air.
Don't do that again.
Look at that little shit Lucrezia with her devious grin.

32.

This morning, when I got into Ward 77, I saw a uniformed police officer in the corridor,
that means there's a patient who needs police supervision.
He is an inmate, brought during the night from Marassi prison because he was too aggressive. He's bound to the bed, huffing like a steam train, covered in gashes and tattoos.
I move with the usual calm, like everything is completely normal.
In the kitchen I think, where the hell do I work? We take in people who even prison can't handle.

Who are we? God's hammer?

33.

Giulia, you are too beautiful to be a psychologist.
How can a person talk to you about their desires
if, just by looking at you, he is assailed by a new one
of such force that he falters in mind and step.
Looking at you, who can still recall their old desires?

34.

Today a young doctor arrived, specializing in Psychiatry. We were expecting him.
He'll be an intern on Ward 77 for a year.
I saw him coming toward me, and I thought:
I'm ruined.
Look how young and confident he is.
My chances with Giulia are ruined.

Youth is a magnet, young people always stick together.
Beautiful young women go out with insignificant young men, who have neither a profession nor wealth, who are boorish, clumsy, ill-mannered,
who don't even know how to speak,
who have nothing other than the future.
Tons, miles, millennia of future.

In the meantime he has walked the three steps to arrive in front of me,
and introduces himself—My name is Marcello.
I shake the hand of my own ruin.

35.

And this is the case for you too, Margherita, my daughter:
to grow up you must learn to tell me to go to hell.
Just don't learn too quickly.

36.

I go into the doctors' room and introduce Marcello to my colleagues.

Rufo, elegant and perfumed, gives a speech on the dignity of Psychiatry,
on the responsibility of the doctor and the sanctity of the therapeutic relationship.
Once he has finished, he dabs his lips with an immaculate handkerchief
and I whisper to Marcello—Don't trust this man.

Edoardo, badly dressed and bewildered, speaks critically of Psychiatry, complaining about the patients,
stuttering, he suggests changing specialty because this one is short on job satisfaction.
Once he has finished, which we know only because he has stopped talking and is gazing out of the window, I whisper to Marcello—This one you can trust.

37.

Rufo, seeing you drag three full doctor's bags around,
anyone would think you were constantly moving house.
You ask for help from whomever you meet, giving yourself a break.
But what have you got in there?
Glasses, prescription pads, Pharmacology manuals, three mobile phones, a blood pressure monitor, a neurological hammer,
an ophthalmoscope, syringes, pills, bandages, enemas,
if I dig deeper I'll also find a pair of forceps and little glass jars of leeches.

Rufo, the only tool you know how to use is the blood pressure monitor,
unburden yourself of this dead weight.
For this job you could be naked and you'd still have everything you need.

38.

Of course Edoardo understands the bipolar patients better than I do
and can see through all their tricks and masks.
He has experienced what it means since boyhood:
to get up, make breakfast and tie your shoelaces alone while your mother is sleeping,
be forgotten at the school gates, to walk home alone
and wait for hours in the rain for someone to open the door,
to not eat in the evening because no one has cooked,
to talk to someone who can laugh and cry in the same breath, to be made to wear a yellow suit to mass on a Sunday,
to hear operatic arias sung all night,
to bump into strange men coming out of your mother's bedroom,
to see your father immobile
sitting with his face in his hands all evening.
When it comes to understanding bipolar patients, Edoardo has at least twenty years on me.

And when the head physician declares in a meeting that there's no such thing as madness,
Edoardo gets up and leaves.

39.

I am here in Intensive Care visiting
a woman who has jumped from the fifth floor.
I am trying to reach her
somewhere.
I still don't know where, nor how, nor when.

Rufo, I'd wager that this morning
though you are flying to Prague, I am traveling further.

40.

Giulia, every time you suffer in life you learn something, encountered by others in the past and that others in the future are yet to encounter.
The beauty of this profession is that all our experiences, however rotten or unspeakable or wretched, will come in useful sooner or later.
Life to a psychiatrist is like a pig to a butcher: nothing goes to waste.

41.

To become a psychiatrist you don't need a reference from the notary, the priest, or the deputy mayor.
To become a psychiatrist you don't need to be intelligent, sensitive, or talented.
To become a psychiatrist, all you need is to have a parent or grandparent who's a bit mad, even the tiniest bit,
and to care about them.
The mad are our siblings. The only difference between us and them is a successful roll of the dice

—the last of a million identical rolls—
that's how we get to be on the other side of the desk.

42.

Carmelo, you checked into Ward 77 during the night, and you come to complain that out of twenty beds
ten are occupied by Moroccans, Senegalese, Ecuadorians, Filipinos, and Sri Lankans.
With a solemn voice you point out that this is not the environment one expects to find when, like you, one admits himself for profound interior suffering.
Then you limp away, with the grave expression of someone who has just done the right thing.
But, Carmelo, did you not admit yourself as a way to hide from the police?
Yes, you clarify with a steady voice, but I was born and raised in Molo.
Ah, an aristocrat.

43.

Accompany me to the Emergency Room, Marcello.
Then I'll find out who you are, I think to myself.

We find three patients in three neighboring rooms.
The first one's whole body is trembling. What's happening? I ask. He doesn't respond. He doesn't even look at me.
I place a hand on his shoulder and the tremor moves into my arm.
The second is stiff as wood. He doesn't speak.
I touch him and try to move his hands, he grabs me by the shoulders and shakes me.

The third is immobile, but his body is relaxed. He doesn't speak. I sit down next to him.
He sighs. I sigh. He shakes his head, I shake my head. I cough, he coughs.

Urgent pain can't be expressed in words,
it is expressed in the body:
it takes three or four days before we can speak to the patient.

Marcello understands immediately. When we leave, he exclaims: Emergency Psychiatry is like a dance!
And he laughs—who wants to dance with me?
The younger nurses turn around and, some out loud, some with a smile, respond—me!
They don't even lower their eyes.

44.

I pay a compliment to Gaia, a nurse, and she says:
Milone, but really, from you who are so naive.
Naive, me, why?
Because you're the only one who doesn't have work lovers, everyone knows it, you big softy.
It only takes me a few days, Gaia, to notice the exchanges between work lovers,
despite myself, I understand when two people fight, when they break up, and when they get back together.
And this is how your relationships are, Gaia.
I, some time ago, spent a year and a half living with a nurse from this department, and nobody ever knew. Call me naive.
And I suppose I was truly naive, because, that nurse, I married her.

45.

Since the dawn of time, nurses have made use of their patients' work to get themselves favors, discounts, benefits of some sort or other:
if the patient is a greengrocer they get some fresh vegetables, if he sells wine, they get a demijohn sent to their house, if he's a lawyer, they ask for an opinion,
if he's a traffic warden, they get their fines cleared.
But what can I say about Mario who, the day after Gloria the prostitute is admitted, pays her a visit.

46.

Walking toward the entrance of Ward 77, we are like fishermen going to sea:
before boarding our boats and leaving the shore, we check the weather forecast.
Calm, slight, moderate, rough.
Storm on its way.
At the door we stop and pull on our wax jackets in the wind.

Chapter Two
The wisteria room

1.

I've found my magic room.
It's a private room, only I have the key.

2.

The room is neither too warm nor too cold,
it is not too near or too far,
opening the door, in the shade of the wisteria,
is not too easy or too hard.
In this room, tucked away around a corner,
we are not in the world, nor are we outside it.
I think it's good for you, Gina.
You are quiet. More silent than the humming lamp
and the gurgling radiator.

I wonder if you have been coming here for three months
just for the smile you glimpsed the first time,
when you entered like a slow gush of air,
and lifted your gaze onto me.
Do you not want anything more than that smile, Gina?
Will you make it last forever?
After all, I too am only here for the smile

that I glimpsed, the first time,
when you entered like a slow gush of air,
and lifted your gaze onto me.

What did we say in that moment, what did we promise each other, so that now we are contented with the silence?

3.

I receive people by the hour,
giving secret appointments,
I make them comfortable,
in the half-light,
we tell each other intimate things,
they receive comfort,
they return home happier
and when they speak to their spouses, they think of me.
Sara, streetwalker, I guess my work and yours are part of the same family.

4.

Do not speak to me in new, modern, newborn words,
which crawl, sneak in everywhere
and end up where they should not be.
Do not speak to me in old, grand, important words,
which sound like they mean a lot but in fact say nothing.
Do not speak to me in the words of others, just heard and swiftly learned,
I get distracted and look out the window
more interested in the croaking of frogs.
Do not speak to me in any words that are not yours.

I will welcome them like dear guests arriving late to a party,
I'll bash the rain off their coats, take their umbrellas and sit them down in the drawing room.

5.

Enrica, you apologize when you come and when you go,
you apologize when you talk and when you're quiet,
you apologize when you do someone a favor and when they tread on your toes,
you apologize because you breathe, because you take up space, because you are alive.
Enrica, whatever did you do that was so bad?

6.

Mr. F, I don't know you, you telephone for an urgent appointment, you say it's a question of life or death,
then you don't turn up;
you call again for a second urgent appointment,
you repeat that it's a question of life or death,
and again you don't turn up.
You call again, I tell you—that's enough, try someone else.
I'm sorry I'll never know what your question of life or death was, Mr. F.

7.

It is me and you, Gina, one across from the other, quiet.
In the silence of the room, my intestine starts to stutter. Yours responds in a shrill voice and ends with an interrogative.

I didn't understand the question, but my intestine answers, varying its tone from high to low, and points something out to finish.
Yours agrees.
Today, Gina, our intestines understand each other better than we do.

8.

You told me—When you talk, Paolo, I don't understand you. For me two plus two makes four, but in your world it can make five or even six.
This war of numbers is the reason we split up.

After twenty years, by chance, we meet on the street. You're still beautiful. One look was enough.
You wanted to tell me that you now understand how two plus two can make five or even six,
and I wanted to tell you that I now understand why two plus two always just makes four.

9.

Lara, you come to me just to tell me that you don't want to come, and this is the last time you'll be coming.
You always come, the most punctual of all my patients.
You always come, to tell me you won't be coming again.

10.

The wisteria room is peaceful.
I hear the tree in the garden swaying in the wind

I hear one dog bark, and another respond
I hear the creak of the Righi funicular, far away on the hillside
I hear a greeting between women at the window.

Faint, quiet
I hear the neighbor above turning on the shower—at this time?
I hear a telephone ring—where?

Faint, quiet
I hear the hum of the fan whirring in the room
and the stubborn slap of the curtain against the glass.

From memory I hear
the coruscating crackle of the fire in the hearth
as the crows caw in the white winter,
and the shouts of children by the sea in the summer light.
Then I look at you, Gina,
silent in front of me

the only thing I can't hear is your voice.

11.

Emilio, you are endlessly sure of yourself.
If I ask how you are, you respond, Very well.

Today, Emilio, you shouted at me—What kind of a doctor are you?
When I tell you I'm well you worry and increase my dose.
When I tell you I'm not well, you're happy and lower my dose.
What kind of a doctor are you?

12.

Lucrezia, for a week you've been calling me four times a day, you leave me a note three times a day, you knock on my door twice a day,
asking me to urgently certify in writing that you are absolutely sound of mind.
Lucrezia, it is the persistence with which you are asking that prevents me from doing it.

13.

Luciano, each time we meet you seek confirmation that I too have been depressed,
else you won't calm down, you won't speak, you won't listen to me and you eye me with suspicion.
Yes, yes, Luciano, I can understand you: I too have been depressed.

But, I wonder—I see people who are schizophrenic, anorexic, addicted to drugs, addicted to sex,
suicidal, homicidal.
How on earth do I do it?

14.

Chiara, you're currently out of work
and you are ashamed
and afraid the neighbors will notice.
So in the morning you pretend you are not home,
you move around quietly in slippers, keep the windows closed,
you don't turn on the radio, or the TV.

In the building there are children screaming,
a housewife talking, an old man on the telephone,
a student running late to college saying hello on the stairs.
You eat without clinking your cutlery and leave your dishes in the sink.
The afternoon is long in the company of the ticking clock.
You wait.

At five o'clock, the elevators start moving, doors slamming, dogs barking, the building refills. Your children return from school.
It's time to clock off. Another day's work done.

15.

Marcello, you meet Emilio at the bar and he offers you a drink.
Do you want my advice? Accept the drink, sure,
but I wouldn't take a ride in his white Porsche:
he does ninety on the Aurelia highway;
nor would I go into business with him to take over that hotel in South Africa: he talks with other people's money;
don't buy it when he tells you this weekend you'll sail to Portofino on his boat: he's a cleaner on the pier;
and don't follow him when he goes to pursue the two women in the back room: he's cocky but he still has to pay them.
It's you who'll have to settle the bill.
Marcello, there's only one thing you can do with Emilio: tell him to go back on his anti-manic meds.

16.

Lucrezia, you've been calling me three times a day for three months,
to make sure I'm alive.
Lucrezia, continue like this and you will kill me.

17.

Lucrezia, you call me at midnight
because you have nocturnal anxieties.
Lucrezia, your nocturnal anxieties are stopping me from sleeping.

18.

Lucrezia, you call me at two in the morning
to tell me that you're scared of throwing yourself out of the window.

In the commotion, my wife wakes up—It's your fault, you're too weak!
Now I'm caught between two fires.
Lucrezia knows that my wife gets angry, and withdraws in an orderly fashion.

19.

Lucrezia, you've been calling me three times a day for three months,
to make sure that you are alive.

Lucrezia, I'm coming there now and I will kill you.

20.

I am at friends' for dinner, the wine is good,
their son asks me what I do.
I explain: I'm a kind of fireman.
I'm called in when someone is so unwell that they can't remember their own name.
They are so unwell they can't say where they come from, nor what has happened to them.
They are so unwell that they don't understand where they are.
These people are lost, like in a fire or out at sea, and I go and find them.
How do you do it?
I improvise.

But how? Don't you have protocols in Psychiatry? his father asks from the kitchen.
Yes, but the patient needs someone who is surprised,
someone who is moved,
someone who will clean up his shit and get back up laughing,
someone who gets confused, who runs away, who puts his hands on him.
He's looking for you, he needs you, not protocols. He's looking for the medic not the medicine.
Now Marco's little face is smiling in admiration.

It would be nice if it was like that.
The truth is that most of them get better on their own, and they come in search of medicine not a medic. There are very few, Marco, who want to play with you.

21.

In the early years I thought you drove a Vespa with your arms, then I learned, you drive it with your ass.
You simply push the seat to one side, horizontally, and the Vespa instantly follows your movement.
In the early years I also thought you drove life with your head.

22.

I know how to do things that I don't know how to describe.
Others know how to describe things that they don't know how to do.

23.

Thank God Lucrezia is coming at four o' clock,
without me saying anything she'll know that I'm down today
and she'll come up with something to raise my spirits.
I just need to wait until four.

24.

Lucilla, on your first visit you bawl your eyes out for an hour,
huge tears furrowing down your cheeks,
describing, one by one, the worst misfortunes that can happen to a human being on this Earth, and from the tenderest age.
Then you do not come to our appointments for an entire month,
but you call me every evening and sob.

Lucilla, I can't award you the trophy for being the sickest patient of my life after a single visit,

there are people who have been working toward that goal
with highly sophisticated methods
for many years.

25.

Roberto, lifeguard from Imperia, you have been taught
to see when someone is thrashing around in need of help,
to get to the person in danger as quickly as possible,
to reassure them, calm them down if they fight,
bring them to the shore,
resuscitate them.

Roberto, now that I'm in this room, out at sea,
drinking salty water,
thrashing around with Filippo who has hold of me and wants to drag me under,
I surmise that you have been taught more than I have.

26.

I don't know why, but once in their lifetime
euphorics have to go and see the Pope.
A person's diagnosis can even be traced back to which religious figure they visit:
no euphoric goes to a priest, a bishop, or a cardinal,
those are sought by the hysterics, the anxious, the depressed, and the schizophrenics,
euphorics skip the lower rungs of the ladder
going directly to the Pope.
The euphorics talk to God, or act in His name:
to them the Pope is just a sane colleague.

*

They set off from all four corners of the earth in flocks, small groups, crowds, and head for Rome by any means possible.
The majority get lost along the way:
they get admitted, robbed,
board the wrong train, disembark at the wrong stop,
run into a tree, fall into a ditch,
forget why they left, fall in love, get drunk;
many others get lost in Rome, or are brought to a halt before the colonnade by a last-minute fear of God.
One of mine left home at night in his Ferrari, and in less than three hours was in St. Peter's Square: God must have had one hand on the car roof along the highway.
Another set off at night by bicycle,
who knows why it's always at night—they're impulsive—
and found himself under the dome of the Vatican after three days pedaling,
cheerfully holding his bike, covered in poop and pee.

As for me, on the rare occasions that I go to Rome and find myself in St. Peter's Square, I scan the crowd for them
and imagine the Swiss Guards, used to it by now—
Stop there, where are you going?
I'm going to give the Pope some advice.

27.

Ines, you live alone. When you turn out the lamp at night, you think—
Maybe tonight's the night.
So, before getting into bed, you make sure to tie up the trash, wash the dishes, fold your clothes and straighten the house:

if it should happen, you wouldn't want anyone to think you were untidy.
You take care to wear a matching pair of socks without holes, knickers that aren't frayed and a clean T-shirt.
Only then do you turn out the light and try to sleep.

28.

Arianna, when I greeted you at the door to my office, I smiled.
From that smile you deduced that I loved you and that we would marry, we'd make love and have a child, then we would start to fight, we'd be unfaithful, we'd request a divorce.
Arianna, you have just sat down, for the first time, on the armchair,
but between us it's already over.

29.

Giulia, try saying "I'm fine" with varying intonations. The meaning becomes, in turn:
I'm fine, I'm unwell, I don't know how I am, mind your own business, I hate you, I love you.
Now try saying "I'm unwell."

30.

Pina, you're a little old lady and you live alone. You have been closed up in your house for two weeks, delirious and hallucinating, in a full psychotic flare-up. Of the neighbors who take care of you, one is out of town, the other is in hospital.

It's August, if we leave you alone you risk not getting to September. We're coming to your house to bring you in.
You don't want to come, but there's not much you can do faced with two adult men.

We are so sure of ourselves that we haven't even called the ambulance and we put you in the car, a white Panda like any other.
From the back seat you mumble your insults and curses.
We stop at a traffic light and a police car rolls up next to us, with the windows open
And you, ungrateful, shout: They're kidnapping me, help!
The officer orders: Pull over and turn off the engine.
The traffic stops.
One of the officers gets out: What's going on here?
I am a doctor and I am taking the lady to the hospital.
I don't want to go, she says.
Are you the son of the lady? No. Are you her guardian? No.
Do you have a warrant to perform an involuntary hospitalization? No.
Doctor, you can't just drive elderly women around the city as and when you please. This is abduction. Where does that leave us?

I'd smack myself in the head.

31.

I am here, bare as God made me
—anyone who wants to, can aim straight for my heart.
A shot, a hit.
Lucrezia, don't take advantage.

32.

Andrea, you have just come into the office.
You are still scanning the room to check I haven't moved anything.
You haven't yet said or done anything.
Yet I, Andrea, could already smash your face in.

33.

Five of us arrive to take you to the hospital.
You have filled your house with garbage, the landing, the stairs.
You don't let us in, we have to kick down the door. We walk on a layer of trash a foot thick.
You lock yourself in the bathroom and turn the tap on, shouting.
We force open the bathroom door.
You weigh three hundred pounds, Luisa, you hold fast to the doorjamb shouting and snarling like a bear. It's hard to pull you out of there.
We start taking slaps, pushes, scratches, you need to be sedated.
There are five of us, but as space is tight only two can work.
You roll yourself up on the floor, it takes us half an hour to give you an injection.
After twenty minutes no effect,
you stare at us with daring in your eyes.
You chant and shout the whole time, happy to see us struggling.
The neighbors start opening their doors, one argues with us because he wants to free you, we tell him, with choice words, to get out, and he phones a lawyer and the police to report us.
Another struggle for a second injection. Nothing.
Useless arguments for another half hour.
When we really start to get angry, you, slowly, surrender.
We manage to drag you down the stairs and push you into

the car, before the small group of protesting neighbors and passersby.
In the Emergency Room you throw stretchers against the walls, six of us have to jump on you and bind you to the gurney.
Finally on Ward 77 we can unrestrain you from the gurney and re-restrain you to the bed,
now you are happy to spit at us and insult and curse our mothers and children.

The following day, I stop by to see how you're doing.
You tell me, through tears: You made me leave my house
with odd slippers on!

34.

Lucrezia, I let you into the wisteria room because I care about you, but now tell me: Where has my little lead soldier on horseback gone, the one from Austerlitz?
It was in my cabinet and now it's not.
Yes I have many of them: I collect them.
It's not true that it was broken: it was injured, he was missing an arm on purpose.
It wasn't worth less: it was worth more.
No of course I don't have proof: but we both know who did it.
You want something of mine? In that case, I give you a gift, you don't steal it from me.
It wasn't stolen: it was borrowed? And what are you going to do, nurse him and give the horse something to eat?

35.

Gina, you see me and you don't see me,

you listen to me and you don't listen to me,
you are here and you're not here.
Gina, I, for you, exist and I don't exist.
This room exists and doesn't exist,
the world outside exists and doesn't exist.

On account of spending time with you, little by little I also start to question everything around me:
fortunately, by the window, the great and old wisteria,
planted before the house was built, is always there,
with its sweet green leaves and plentiful lilac flowers,
still and motionless.

While there is the wisteria, Gina, you can't fool me.

36.

Cesare, stop giving antidepressants to all the Genoese people you meet.
It's true, the Genoese complain a lot, but they are not depressed.
You, coming from Rome, need to learn differential diagnosis.

The mumble has rules, it's pop music.
It's a layman's blues, talking of the struggle of man
but not seeking salvation.
It's a self-absorbed blues, because it says: Things are going badly for me, I can't do anything for you.
It's a lying blues: when a Genoese complains of something
it means he already has the answer in his pocket.
Complaining is a frugal way of celebrating victory.
If a Genoese is truly unwell, he doesn't complain, he goes quiet.

The lament of the depressive has a unique beat, repetitive, heavy.

It says: This is nothing to do with you, but in some way it's your fault.
The mumble is liberatory: we are united against someone, we are in the same boat.
The music is different, you can hear it from the first syllable.

If someone is not from Genoa
and they try to find a solution to the problem,
the Genoese pulls back.
He'll leave without saying a thing.

37.

I don't enter at night on tiptoes,
it is they who come in the light of the sun.
Sometimes, in ten minutes, I have opened the safe.
I rob intimacy, but don't overdo it.
I am a gentleman robber.

38.

And after a whole week listening to the problems of my patients,
on Sundays at last I can listen to the problems of my friends.

Chapter Three
Lucrezia

1.

You sit down and don't speak.
You know that in hospital I can't stand silence,
I can't make myself shut up.
In order to stay quiet I dig my nails into my skin, tap my feet, I look like I'm desperate to pee.
I can't do it, I give up and ask you: So, how are you doing?
You say nothing, you smile, you win.
Lucrezia, in a silence race with you, I will always lose.

2.

At this time in the evening my face is tired.
I've run out of smiles, whines of approval, throat-clearing, sighs, the looks of incredulity and questioning and, the hardest of all, amazement.
I've even run out of the whistles of admiration, the knitting of my brow, the raising of eyebrows, winks and funny faces with my tongue.
I can scrape together the odd half smile and a dented yawn, but that's not enough: it's time to close up shop.
Lucrezia, come by again tomorrow.

3.

On the ward I am faced with this giant who has cut his wrists and is crying over a lost love, with huge tears that pool on the desk. He wants to leave.
I'm undecided whether or not to keep him by force
—but he's so big! Who would be able to?—
or let him go.
I don't know what to do, and I grumble.
You appear, Lucrezia, at the door, and your eyes and hand signal to let him go.
I calmly follow.

Today is the discharge of a calm and silent gentleman, who is sitting at the window immersed in the leaden November sky.
His daughter has come to collect him.
Greetings, small talk, tinged with sadness.
You appear, Lucrezia, at the door, and your eyes and finger signal no.

Lucrezia's judgment, for me, is Gospel.

4.

You see me by chance in the largest shopping mall in the city, you look at me bewildered.
Lucrezia, it's not Mary or Joseph, it's me.
What are you doing here?
A spot of shopping, I respond, without undermining your amazement.
You watch dreamily as I walk away.

5.

Cecilia, when you arrived in ER you had headphones on
you were up on your feet dancing in the ambulance surrounded
by silence:
the soldiers, out of fear, didn't switch off your music.
You also danced on the stretcher that brought you to Ward 77.
When you entered—it was the first time—
we asked you: What are you listening to?
Reggae!
And us doctors and nurses, in the silence,
all began to dance.

6.

Friday, fritto misto di mare.
Sunday, pasta with pesto, potatoes, and green beans.
Tuesday, ravioli with ragú.
Wednesday, roast meat and potatoes.

Not a day goes by that walking into Ward 77 at a mealtime you aren't greeted by a thousand different fragrances.
It is not for the patients: they are served precooked, odorless stuff that gets brought in, these are the smells of homemade, rustic haute cuisine that shouts out, eat me.
It is the nurses cooking their lunch or dinner.
Early in the morning they arrive laden with grocery bags from the market, put the meat in the fridge, vegetables on the worktop, set down braids of warm bread,
they put the white wine in the fridge, the red in the pantry
and the green and black olives in separate cups.
Throughout the day, between one job and another, they nip into the kitchen to wash vegetables,

chop carrots, boil eggs, slice bread and spread butter.
If you call a nurse, he'll leave the kitchen with his hands covered in flour: he was rolling the gnocchi.

7.

I walk around the ward on tiptoes, like a hunting cat.
I intercept a secret meeting between Lucrezia and Carmelo.
What do a young girl and a sly old drug addict have to discuss?
They are talking about how to use razor blades, and I understand that they have one ready for a practical demonstration.
You hold it with two fingers like this, no you hold it with three fingers like that.
In hospital you cut like this, in jail you cut like that.
A razor blade master class.

I am about to intervene,
when Carmelo asks her where on earth she hides them,
so I stop and prick up my ears.
but she changes the subject: Do you know how to make the knot to hang yourself?
At this point I intervene.
Carmelo, stop leading this girl astray!
Me, doc? It's her leading me astray.
I didn't doubt it.

8.

When we admit Lucrezia, her mother is often seen outside the ward.
She doesn't ring to enter or ask for news:
she sits silently, curled into herself,

after an hour or two she gets up and leaves.
She told me that a mental illness kept her far away from her daughter, in white rooms under neon lights.
A thing inside her head, she told me.
Her fears distracted her from the fears of Lucrezia, her insecurity stifled her voice, her sight, and her actions.
For years she has chosen to keep herself away from her,
to do her less harm.
When she discovered that her daughter suffered like her, she couldn't help trying to get closer to her, but Lucrezia wasn't listening anymore.
I lost the match, she says.
And who raised Lucrezia?
She was put into the care of her paternal grandparents but she was never very fond of them, nor were they of her.
She was the brightest girl in her class, she was well-liked, her schoolmates' parents would invite her round to study and then have dinner,
then, hearing her story, they would invite her to spend the night.
There were three or four families who contended for her.
After high school, something collapsed.
In a matter of months she was no longer herself.
Now she lives with friends in the city center, but nobody knows precisely who with or where.

May I ask, madam, who is looking after you?

9.

The good and the bad that we do to another person reverberates and propagates in a thousand ways
among their relatives, friends, and acquaintances
and, over time, it is transmitted to all their descendants.

It might be something microscopic, a movement of atoms,
a shadow, a shudder, but it exists and it spreads through the universe.
You see, Giulia, we contribute to bettering or worsening the universe,
and, for this, we have a responsibility.

10.

I phone Lucrezia's father.
I'll come tomorrow, he assures me. He doesn't come.
After three calls, three agreements, and three absences,
he turns up drunk.
He notices the bitterness in my eyes and mumbles:
I haven't always been like this.

How many times have I told Lucrezia to come and live with me . . .
She doesn't want to, I observe.
But if only she wanted to . . .
She doesn't want to!

11.

Alessandro, since your wife died at eighty
—you have two winters more—
you packed your suitcase and put it under your bed.

Every morning you open your eyes
and marvel that you are still here.

12.

Lucrezia in ER for an overdose!
The time it takes to get there breathless and they're already pulling you out of it by the hair with intravenous drugs.
Stupid girl! A thousand times stupid! This is the last thing we need.
Who gave them to you? You say nothing.

The next time I see Carmelo, I'll wring out his balls.

13.

Marcello, don't give a patient you don't know a drug that has just been launched. How can you evaluate the effect of it?
You have to know one of them, the medicine or the patient.
You respond: But Rufo gave three new drugs to the new admission!
Try to find the reason on the atlas: conferences in Vienna, Athens, and Madrid.

14.

It is sad, Lucrezia, to find you one day arguing out loud with nobody.
You protest, retort, apologize, insult with such fervor.
Alone in the room.
You are the prosecutor who offends and makes threats
stamping your feet on the ground, your hair a mess,
then you are the victim spreading your arms wide weeping and sobbing.

But this is a task for me, I'll increase your meds.

Don't worry: I'll bring out the big guns.

15.

The other day, at dinner with friends, my daughter says to me: I don't understand how you make a living. How many mad people can there be in this city?
Let's see, I say, let's count how many there are in this building. How many apartments are there in total?
Twenty, she responds.
O.K., and how many mad people can you think of?
There's just the crazy guy on the third floor, the one who talks to himself.
So we have one schizophrenic. Now tell me, isn't there a drug addict somewhere?
Yes, on the first floor.
Could there be a very thin girl, so thin she looks like a skeleton?
Giovanna, on our floor.
Is there anyone who can be found, morning and night, cradling a glass of white wine at the bar? Yes, Giorgio, fifth floor.
We couldn't have done without an alcoholic.
Now I want to know, is there a man with a gaunt face
who hardly goes out, never opens his door,
deadly silent and doesn't even venture out onto his pigeon dropping-encrusted balcony?
Yes, Silvio, on the third floor. Paranoid, check.
Let's move on to the depressives. Have you ever heard a neighbor say: We're not going to the beach, my wife is in bed?
Yes, top floor.
Just the one depressive? Let's pretend that's so.
And we'll close with Alzheimer's: you're not going to tell me that in this whole building there's not a single little old lady who jabbers on and on and throws things out of the window?

Well actually there are two.
You see, if all of them were to be treated, I'd make my living from this building alone.

16.

The tailor sees everyone as badly dressed,
the hairdresser, everyone disheveled,
the milliner, everyone hatless,
the physiotherapist, everyone injured,
and I, psychiatrist, see everyone as mad.

17.

The nurse puts her mouth close to my ear and whispers:
Lucrezia is nowhere to be seen, she's not in her room or in the toilet.
Uh-oh! It's nighttime and we set off room by room with flashlights, so as not to wake everyone.
We find you in the recently-admitted eighteen-year-old's bed, sweet girl, daughter of lawyers.
You are both naked. My first impulse is to split you up, but then I see you in the light:
you are sleeping like babies, your young faces, one next to the other.
Two little girls.
I've never seen you so peaceful.
Neither of you have contagious illnesses . . .
I whisper to the nurses: Go, go, we'll let them sleep.
The nurses look at me. I said: Go.
Tomorrow we'll dismiss one of them,
but for now, we'll let them sleep.

18.

Best to keep your eyes always open on the ward.
I realize that at the end of the corridor a patient is inviting Lucrezia into the men's bathroom. Lucrezia enters.
I get up and start walking toward them ready to raise my voice, when I hear a thud and a moan of pain,
I start running.
I bump into Lucrezia calmly leaving the bathroom, she smiles at me: What's up, doc?
I look inside. The man is losing blood from his nose, holding onto the sink and complaining: She took twenty euros, I want my money back.
Did she sign the bank note? I ask. You thank heaven that everything is over here.

19.

Sometimes, Lucrezia, you give me such a sense of solitude that, as soon as our session is over, I have to call my wife;
if she doesn't pick up, my daughter; if she doesn't pick up, a friend.
I say: It's me, and then I don't know how to say why I called.

20.

On Monday morning as soon as I set foot on the ward and am told,
among other notices,
as if it were nothing:
ah, Lucrezia is bound to the bed.
Lucrezia! Why?

She spent the whole weekend fighting with Rufo, who was on call, and last night he restrained her.

Unbind her! Then send Rufo to see me!
Doc, before unbinding her, go and see her.
I enter her room. The bands around her wrists and ankles have never horrified me so much.

How are you? You slowly open your eyes and look at me with a gaze full of hatred.
Lucrezia, I wasn't here Saturday and Sunday: they're my days off.
Now listen to me: If I unbind you, will you be good?
You emit the roar of a wild beast.

21.

A sleepless night is scant for consoling yourself over the day before.
A sleepless night is scant for preparing yourself for the day to come.
Harsh is the morning: the drawers are reopened and the knives resurface.

22.

We got Lucrezia onto a supported employment program. After a week she suggests an improvement to a procedure that is accepted, the office manager smiles at her.
An employee, who has worked there for years, is envious and gives her a hard time
and remarks in public upon her every fault.
Lucrezia endures it, until one day she shouts: Shut up! You ugly

old idiot! And dress a bit better why don't you, always wearing that red skirt that makes you look like an ape!

All true, but it was up to us to find her another office.

23.

Lucrezia likes the work: I get out of the house, she says, I talk to people, I learn
and I distract myself from the voice.
The voice is the one that every morning, after she has drunk her coffee, slipped on her shoes and opened the door,
gives her authorization to go to work.
Lucrezia waits, leaning on the handle, for the voice's yes or no.
If the voice says yes, she leaves in a buoyant dash, as if she were off to a party.
If the voice says no, she spends the day at home crying and staring at the wall.
If the voice is unclear, she takes a gamble,
but in the evening when she gets home she pays for it:
the jealous voice will insult and threaten her
until she closes her eyes.
To work, Lucrezia pays double the price.

24.

Lucrezia, you don't come to our sessions when you're unwell because the voice forbids you.
When you do come, the voice forbids you from talking about certain things.
I realize this when you do not respond to a question and look up at the ceiling,

so I too look up at the ceiling, then at you: you nod.
It becomes clear, there are three of us in here.

The fact is that if you go home the voice will stop you from taking your meds, so now: either I admit you
or I give you a depot injection that will last a month.
Neither you, nor I, nor the voice likes either of these options.
But it needs to be decided now.

25.

You were seen in a deserted church, early in the morning, on a bench looking around.
So I ask, Lucrezia: Do you believe in God?
You look at me bewildered.
For you every crucifix genuinely bleeds,
when you look at Saint Sebastian you feel the arrows enter flesh,
you cannot pray because the gaze of God is real and terrorizes you.

I would like to say to you: Lucrezia, first heal, then believe.
But for you who never heal,
caught between need and fear, all that remains is to try to believe.
It is easy to believe for sane people, who believe in nothing.

26.

I am discharging you for the fourth time and I try once more:
Wouldn't you be better off in a Therapeutic Community?
There would be lots of other young people, and lots of support workers. I'll continue to see you, I promise.
I've told you a thousand times: I want to live on my own.

I smile.
Don't even try it with your smiles, doc, stop trying to trick me: if you force me to go, I'll set fire to the Community.
O.K., Lucrezia, let's talk about this again later.

27.

How mild this spring. You are calm, your voice has disappeared, but I wasn't expecting this other surprise from you:
I went up to Palazzo Tursi for your wedding,
you told me last week.
You are marrying a Tunisian, he arrived by boat a short time ago, younger than you. Handsome as a flower, curly hair, always smiling.
You are happy, glowing, in your salmon pink dress.

There are few of us. I recognize Carmelo and another two drug addicts,
I greet two patients who were admitted some months ago, then there's a priest and a nun, and another dozen people, very ordinary, that I don't know.
I can't see your parents. Two beautiful, elegant women stand out, affectionate toward you, I imagine they are your high school friends, one is your witness.
When you come out we throw rice, and an accordion plays.

Are you leaving already, doc?
Yes, congratulations Lucrezia, from the bottom of my heart.
Doc . . .
Yes.
If I wanted to have a child, should I stop treatment?
Ah, well . . . the lithium should be suspended, the rest lowered . . . but we would need to talk about it.

Look at you! That face! Don't worry:
I won't live long, I can't have a child.

28.

Emilio, do you truly believe that when you die
the mountains will crumble,
the earth will crack,
and the moon, the sun, and the stars will cease to shine?
Emilio, believe me:
Not a single ant will deviate from its path,
not a single wave in the sea its wash,
not a grain of sand
will notice your departure.

29.

I saw you again, Lucrezia: you are in a hurry.
You're in a hurry to heal, a hurry to love, a hurry to understand,
a hurry to live.
You are irritated with me for being so slow, so stupid.
You say to me: Stop smiling all the time! You help me.
But what are you frightened of missing?

30.

You rush in from outside the hospital sobbing
about those who don't love you, about destiny, about the world.
I smile at you, I don't know what I say and I leave you with one
of us, then I return, you have dried your nose,
our gazes meet across the room,

you mumble something, your eyes still shining,
you say thank you and leave.
I bid you farewell with just my hand.
The world, Lucrezia, is the same as before.

31.

Why don't I want to go to the hospital today?
Why does the journey seem so long?
Why are the cars moving so slowly?
And why are the children on their way to school and the mothers with their strollers so beautiful?
Why would the rising sun call me far away?
But I am already on the tree-lined path.

32.

Today as I walked onto the ward, I was accosted by three colleagues.
Someone told me, Lucrezia, that you ran away from the ward in the night and boarded the 35.
Someone told me that you got off at the end of the line and climbed up onto the city wall.
Someone must have told me that you walked toward the balustrade and threw yourself off.
Another repeated it: Lucrezia threw herself off.
Another told me: Don't take it like that. Sit down. You did everything you could.

At that point, somebody asked me if I could swap shifts.

33.

I know, Marcello, the first suicide is the worst.
At first it is shock, even if the patient had shown us in countless ways that she would kill herself.
Can you die just like that? When you are young, death is such a distant thing.
Then it is pain.
When you are young you become fond of the patients in a different way. It is as if the dead person were a relative, a friend.
We cry. We get angry.
What did I do wrong? What did I forget to do?
We would like to go to the funeral, but we are ashamed, as if we are the guilty ones.
For three days we can't work.
That's how it is, Marcello, the first time.

34.

When the people of Genoa are sad and bruised, they climb up onto a clifftop and talk to the sea.

The sea is there for you, it doesn't hide,
when you speak it doesn't interject.
With the sea you can cry, shout, swear,
throw rocks, it doesn't get scared.
It continues going, back and forth:
seeking you, not seeking you,
calling you, not calling you.
It would be nice to learn the secrets of the sea.

The sea is immense, it is everything.
In its presence, there is no pain that doesn't seem small.

Facing the sea you rediscover your place in the world and in time,
you see how short life, with its suffering, is,
and you manage to ask yourself the question you fear the most.
The worst is over, let's see what's next.
The sea listens to people one at a time
all the while coming and going:
touching you, not touching you,
taking you, not taking you.

The sea waits, and as soon as the pain starts to feel lighter
it distracts you with a cold wind that slips under your coat or a sun that burns your skin.
It is cunning. It starts to rock you with the rhythm of the wave
that breaks between the rocks and then recedes,
now stronger, now quieter.
And, without you realizing, it bewitches you, hypnotizes you, lulls you to sleep.
Finally you rest.
When it's time, it splashes your feet with water.
You wake up.
You say thank you, goodbye and you leave.

What a master.
Compared to the sea, we psychiatrists are nothing,
we are the tiny puddle cupped between hands
trying to put out a fire.

35.

Ignoring death does not make us immortal.
Neither does thinking about it all the time.
Maybe thinking about it every so often?

36.

I wasn't able to help you, Luciano. You left home one afternoon, you got to the overpass on the Aurelia highway
and took to the air.
When I ride my bicycle, I have to cross that bridge and think:
Now, as punishment, I too will slip and fall.
And the town I come across a little further on is where Giuseppe fell, from the railway bridge.
On my way back into the city, I cycle along the city wall
where Iris flew one month ago.

As the years pass, my carefree trips, between the bougainvillea
and the sea, are transformed into something all too pensive.
This Sunday I won't take my bicycle out from under the stairs.

37.

Luciano, in order to be stronger than pain,
stronger than fear,
stronger than anger,
you have become wind.

38.

But if the failed suicides don't know why they tried to kill themselves,
how can we possibly hope to find out?

Chapter Four
In the city

1.

Alfio, the moment you feared has arrived.
They knock on your front door.
Do they want a showdown?
Why now?
You have done nothing different. You haven't provoked them.
For months you have endured, you haven't rebelled, while they haven't let you out of their sight for a moment, the cameras and microphones hidden in those microscopic holes in the wall (you find new ones every morning).
They knock on the door again. Signor Alfio, open up!
For months you've been locked in your house,
pretending not to exist.
But they knew exactly what you were doing,
through which rooms you were moving.
And so you stayed still all day.
Only a smile, in the evening: Today, too, I have fooled them.
They knock on the door again. Signor Alfio, open up!
You take the big knife from the kitchen.

These are my thoughts as I stand in front of your door, Alfio,
when I hear rummaging and strange sounds from inside.
This is the first home visit, we have never met.
The nurse whispers to me: Let's call the police.

I gesture that we should wait.
You rattle numerous chains for five minutes,
then the door opens.
Darkness, nobody on the other side, just a sort of lament.
We do not move: Good day, Signor Alfio.
Come in.
He is small, he seems harmless.
As soon as we cross the threshold we hear the clamor of the door closing behind us,
a complex system of cables and counterweights,
but there is not just one door, there is another and yet another: it is a triple door.
Eventually everything falls silent, a cable swings.
Alfio observes us with caution:
Nobody can enter or leave now.
The nurse tells me with her eyes: If he doesn't kill you, I will.

2.

Yesterday I heard a war correspondent say that we Europeans are living in a doll's house,
unconscious of the dramas of the world.

I know people who spend the night under shelling in Vico Untoria,
people who in the mornings go down to the trenches in Via Venti Settembre,
people stripped of all their rights in prisons in Salita del Carmine,
people lost in the desert just two hundred meters from the Principe Station.

3.

Genoa is not a squared city, it is a crooked city: there is always a quicker route.
Between my house and the hospital alone there are fifteen shortcuts, each quicker than the next.
When I am with my wife I have to follow her shortcut, else she gets angry,
but I know that mine is quicker.

4.

The most dangerous moment of a home visit
is when the patient offers you coffee.
You try to say no, but they insist, you insist on saying no but they get up to make it anyway.
They open old sideboards
and take out ancient cups that don't match,
dust-covered and discolored, chipped and veined.
They rummage in the bottoms of drawers for tarnished teaspoons of varying lengths.
From a kitchen cupboard comes a stove-top coffee pot that's blacker than coal, they fill it with water from a greasy, dripping tap,
then open a packet of coffee from an Asian brand, no aroma,
and put it on to brew over a broken flame, flickering in and out,
they prepare the sugar, grubby, hard, grey clumps,
and find the courage to smile at you, happy.
Then they ask if you'd like something to eat with your coffee.
You're halfway through saying: No, thank you,
when out of nowhere appear:
dried-up fruit gummies, licorice buttons, chocolate cigarettes,
pastries bought goodness knows when with cream dry like

clotted putty, anise biscotti, stale Pavesini cookies, two marzipan bananas.
The richer ones, around Christmas, serve an Easter cake, which lands on the table like a rock and spins around.
Once the coffee is in the cups, there is a moment of silence and uncertainty.
You wonder for a second: what if they're poisoning me?
Then we smile at one another across the table and dig in.

5.

Walking through the alleys on patient visits,
it's impossible to avoid rubbing up against prostitutes:
the alleys are narrow and their hips are wide,
sometimes they put a chair in the middle of the street,
to lean back and exhibit their legs.

Prostitutes have a psychiatric spirit: if you want to know how a patient is,
ask the woman pulling on stilettos in the doorway or blocking the alley with her enormous buttocks:
nobody knows better than she does.

As she finishes doing up her straps,
she lifts her bust and face toward you
and, for a moment,
she doesn't look like a prostitute
and you don't look like a psychiatrist.

6.

Angelo, you refuse to come to our appointments, so I surprise you at your house.
Your mother opens the door and indicates where you are with desperate eyes.
I walk into the hallway and you hide in your room,
I knock on the door of your room and you pop up in the kitchen.
I take the long way to reach you in the kitchen
and you step back into your room.
I turn back, knock again, and run into the kitchen to catch you out, but you have slipped out the front door
and are gone for a few hours, free and happy,
while I'm there waiting for you like a fool,
until the voice of your mother informs me:
See, he's run away.
I stay a while sipping coffee
and I don't dare look your mother in the eye when she murmurs: But doctor, will you manage, at some point, to stop this imbecile running away?

7.

Giorgio, like every Saturday afternoon, you went to Vico Untoria to fuck old Almira.
She was sick—she is seventy—so they offered you the younger Lidia.
You accepted, but demanded a discount.

8.

End of July. One morning you look outside:

Genoa is deserted.
Did everyone leave in the night?
Immense spaces, emptiness, through the tremble of warm air you can see buildings far away.
Everything is still, like a lizard on the wall.
Silence: the sounds of the sea and the squawking of seagulls reach you on the hillside.
Rare connoisseur tourists searching for something.
But there it is, something is happening: old shutters, closed for months, are opened,
rooms, dark for months, are illuminated,
forgotten locks creak.
This is the moment when Gino, Elisa, Enzo, and the others pluck up the courage,
open their doors and come out onto the street.
They wander along the sidewalks, sit on benches,
talk to themselves at the crossroads, study the traffic lights,
call out to the cats.
Dressed in the strangest clothes, some in anoraks, some in sweaters, some in hiking boots, some in flip-flops.
It is an explosion, like snails after the rain.
The city is all theirs. Rulers for a day.
Scampering about on my Vespa, I notice how few of them I know.
The city is full of people who don't exist.

End of August. Lines of cars, filled with yawning, return from vacation.
In a few days the snails slide back into their holes.
Those who didn't see them, never will.

9.

For fifty years I have walked around Genoa

and I still often chance upon,
less than a mile from my house,
lanes I have not yet followed.
I will die at the end of a life of walking around Genoa, not having walked it all.

10.

Heavy is the earth and heavy is your body, Giuseppina. You never get out of bed.
Since Piero's wedding you haven't opened the wardrobe
where your good shoes lie in the dark.
It takes half an hour to get your slippers on, another half an hour to get you up, then you drag your feet, step by step, and it takes you half an hour to circumnavigate the bed.
You are attached to that bed like a castaway to an island in the sea.
In front of the bed is the large closet.
In the room there is you, the bed, and the large closet.

In the closet lies your mother's wedding dress with the hat from the reception
and the green dress, honeymoon on Lake Como.
In the closet lies your father's railway uniform, stationmaster at Levanto.
There lie the black and white photos of your peasant grandparents leaning against a grapevine
and the hungry faces of your parents during wartime.
There lie the photos of your confirmation in Lagaccio, cocktails at Righi, a schoolmate pulling a funny face.
There lies your teaching certificate and the signature from your first day as a substitute: at the D'Annunzio, you were teaching Pascoli, do you remember?

The class was making noise, paper airplanes were flying through the air,
best blur it out.
There lies the splinted brace that a mean orthopedist wanted to make you wear.
There lies a fake love letter you wrote to yourself,
and the real one you wrote to Piero and never sent.
There lies the little bag of sugar-coated almonds from Piero's wedding, since which he has had three of Giusi's children.
Out of your belly have come ten imaginary children that the Haldol can't undo. You are tired of these pregnancies, with no fathers, no parties, no christenings.

Giuseppina, you sleep opposite your life enclosed in the closet. It is already an Egyptian sepulchral chamber, this room. You are buried alive.
Your ancient mother coughs, the canary chirps in the dining room: I get up, I take my coffee into the kitchen, the stuffy air, I feign interest in the canary,
I agree on how prices are going up, I change your medications arbitrarily, your mother understands and sighs: we'll keep her as she is.
As soon as she opens the door, I leave down the stairs,
finally free.

11.

Giovanna, it's the first time we're going out together.
You look pretty and I'm taking you to dinner at a restaurant in the old town.
It is already dark, we are walking beside the traffic of Via Gramsci.
Suddenly a hulk of a man pops out from a doorway, heavily made-up, all leopard-print, long blond hair,
as soon as he sees me he smiles and says: Ciao Paolo.

And then sashays away.
I've worked with drug addicts for a long time, many of whom are transvestites, the only affectionate ones.

I don't have time to explain, Giovanna:
He walks toward us, high heels, shiny black leather pants, tall and strong with a pink shawl around his shoulders and dark red lips, he looks at me mischievously
and smiles as he gets closer, licking his lips with the tip of his tongue: Ciao Paolo . . .

But the worst is the transvestite who right now, across four lines of traffic on a crowded road, is waving his arms and warbling: Ciao Paolo!

I know, Giovanna, we need to talk.
But where is this darned restaurant.

12.

You will never see them.
You will never hear them.
You will not even suspect their existence.
Yet there are many of them: hundreds, thousands in a city.

They are locked in their rooms.
They survive for years.
If they don't empty their bedpans from the window,
if they don't beat their parents,
if they don't scream at night from the balcony or the landing,
they can stay on their islands for twenty, thirty years, like Robinson Crusoe.

If you go looking for them, they throw arrows, treat you like a cannibal.
If you force them into a corner, they adopt, amid the urine and the filth,
the manner of an English gentleman:
Sorry, is there something the matter?
I've been here a few days, I'm just waiting for the steam train back to England.

13.

Valerio and I went to hunt one of them down.
Difficult work, dangerous and not particularly satisfying.
This work comes up when the parents are dying.
The father is in bed, the mother opens the door with trembling hands. Robinson Crusoe is somewhere, hidden in the forest of his bedroom.
He slips through the house, hunched over, swift, silent.
Then we see him: his beard is untamed, his hair tufty,
fingernails four inches long, hairs coming out of his nose and ears, black teeth, encrusted T-shirt.
He moves quickly, huffs, mumbles, snarls, then uses words.
Mamma, damn woman, why did you let them in?
And the chase begins again. You are my downfall. Damn woman.

I am here and, I don't know why,
but wild boar hunting on Monte Gottero springs to mind,
one stays in place, the other drives him out, whistles, shoots.
I don't even have a gun.

He doesn't reciprocate our greetings, he says he'll report us.
This is my house, what I do with my life is my business, thank you and good day: Mamma, show the gentlemen out.

I too, at this point, would like to say:
thank you and good day to you too,
it's been a pleasure.
And step out into the sunshine to get an ice cream in Castelletto.

14.

To carry out an involuntary hospitalization means to burst into someone's home and forcibly drag them to the hospital.
It's a military operation.
Like all military operations, it requires everyone in the squad to know each other, to trust one another, and to agree on the hierarchy.
What happened at Tommaso's house, Valerio, must never happen again.

In his room, in front of him, I discreetly whisper to you:
let's proceed
and you respond:
no, let's wait.
Wait for what, Valerio? I am the doctor and you are the nurse, what are you suggesting?
That we say to the patient: wait a moment
and you and I go to another room and discuss whether it is fair or not to take Tommaso by force?
Perhaps ask his relatives and neighbors what they think? Put it to a vote? Pull the answer out of a hat?
Valerio, if I am responsible, and I say let's proceed, we proceed.

15.

To be dragged off your island, into the light, after twenty years, is no small thing,

it's a terrifying experience, like being skinned alive.
But there is something that in the end is stronger than terror: curiosity.
After a few days on Ward 77, finally among other people, strange as they may be, these Robinson Crusoes
—secretly—
are spying,
observing, scrutinizing, listening.
They'll never admit it, they'll continue to accuse us of having ruined their lives
but, as soon as we leave the room, they start to enjoy themselves.
Then one day we find them chatting away with another patient.
After twenty years.
We pretend it's nothing, and so do they.

16.

When there's no way of avoiding it and we have to do an involuntary hospitalization,
before setting off,
like warriors donning their armor,
like choosing weapons before a battle,
there is a moment of sacred stillness.
The doctor wonders why he chose this career, wistfully says farewell to his wife and children and gives himself a pep talk.
The nurses pull on their sneakers, change their scrubs for old T-shirts.
A glance at the patient records, where nothing is ever written.
Each person says to the other: don't screw this up.
Each person kisses their lucky charm, wishes for good fortune.
And off they go.

17.

Gino, who's going to get this rowdy patient in a neck hold, you or me?
We can't just stand here: he's throwing punches and breaking everything.
The person who is behind him has to do it, and right now, Gino, you are behind him.
Gino, are you going to do something?

Gino, that you have a stiff neck and cramp in one arm
that the CAT scan found arthrosis in your shoulder,
that you only got into work this morning by the grace of God,
tell me before, next time, not after.

18.

Giusi, old transsexual,
when, with a companion, I pass
the front of the hovel where you wait half-naked on the bed,
don't call out, like you do, in your booming, silky voice,
my first name and surname,
just wave your hand,
no, just blow me a kiss,
no, a smile is sufficient,
no, do nothing,
just think of me.

19.

Marcello, to diagnose someone all you need is to look at their shoes.

The depressives wear slippers or soft shoes and dark, odorless socks. If a depressed person has laces it means there's someone looking after them who ties their shoes, else they're not depressed
or worse, they're a methodical depressive and a high suicide risk.

Euphorics don't have time to waste,
they pull on old boots to save a few seconds then walk around for hours in pain.
Restless euphorics walk day and night.
Their socks are sweaty and fetid, all colors, often mismatched and holey.
If a euphoric turns up in ER in slippers or barefooted, with blackened feet, they need to be admitted.

Schizophrenics sometimes wear mismatched shoes on a whim, a superstitious mockery of the world.
Paranoiacs wear shoes that are good for running in. If they turn up in muddy military boots, they need to be admitted.
The shoes of the homeless are broken, but stiffened by dirt, indestructible.

Neurotics turn up with shiny shoes that squeak on the ground,
I look around, wondering where the noise is coming from.

20.

In the old town of Genoa, the biggest piazzas are the insides of churches, sometimes, the best way to get across the city is to enter through one nave and out through the other.
There are those who go into the church to rest their legs,
to enjoy the cool air, to shelter from the rain,
to hear the music, by mistake.

You, Elio, though, you're strange:
every time you go into a church you think about God.
Does he exist? Does he not exist? What's he like? Why did he create us?
Then you stay ruffled for hours, all chewed up.

21.

The sacristan guides us: Come.
The church is dim and deserted.
As we wander past a side-altar
the baroque angels carefully studying us,
the sacristan lets out a light fart, light and long.
As we wander past Saint George slaying the dragon,
the horse eyeing us up,
the sacristan lets out another fart,
light, long, monotonous.
As we walk in front of a painting, in the style of Caravaggio,
Holofernes observing us,
the sacristan picks up the same note,
syncopated and disjointed this time.
As we walk around a fifteenth-century confessional,
a ghost behind the curtains,
the sacristan completes his opus.
He then opens three doors for us without farting: holding it in for when we arrive in front of the immense tapestry of the Wedding Feast at Cana, now he relieves himself.
And then he shows us into the priest's private apartment.

The priest, all dressed in black, has some tics and a tremble in his hand.
He has various troubles, but the one that he suffers most
is that when he walks into the church

he feels rising within him a strong desire to swear,
he controls it with difficulty,
he lives in the fear of not managing to hold it down,
he is terrified that the heresy will burst out for all to hear,
he strangles a blasphemous thought down the middle,
he regains his composure,
then he starts suffering again.
It's coming, it won't be held back any longer. He rushes out of the church and slowly the tension eases.

Nasty symptom for a priest.
Spectacularly beautiful for a young psychiatrist like me.

22.

Rufo, you have been off work for a week, then you arrive from Rome and boast of having become intimate with an undersecretary who talks every day to the Minister of Health.
Rufo, not to boast, but I, staying in Genoa to work, have become intimate with a guy who talks every day to God.

23.

If exclusively the most intelligent students were accepted to study Medicine,
who would save Psychiatry from ruin?

24.

Lia, your flaky mind is crumbling from dementia.
You welcome us gracefully into your beautiful bourgeois home

on Via Caffaro, show us your paintings, the library, and insist on offering tea. You sit us down on the red armchairs and make us wait forever.
(You sent away the staff, you say, they were stealing).
The marble floors, the old furniture, the grand piano:
your mind wavers but the world around you does not fall apart,
its head mysteriously remains held high.
Modesty, order, dignity, respect.
Indestructible bourgeois decorum is your salvation, Lia.
Finally you come back in, pushing a cart with clinking china cups.
You smile. You pass the cup with shaking hands:
we observe it
as it rises through the cloud of doubt
like how the promontory at Portofino
appears clear and unmoving to the sailor unsure of his route.
The world is not dissolving, only the sugar cube under the teaspoon.
Death itself, when it comes, will have to sit at your little table,
Lia, and delay its task,
to drink, calmly, the tea from the Dutch china.

25.

In certain back streets in the old town of Genoa, medieval skyscrapers rise eight stories high.
The stairs are narrow, heads bowed and shoulders only just making it through.
They are steep, each step a different height.
They twist and turn like intestines in the building's stomach,
with no landings: the doors open onto the stairs
and they do not have numbers or names:
if you're looking for someone, you're on an adventure.

One evening, Livio and I set off with an involuntary hospitalization order for Sergio, a schizophrenic who lives in these streets:
the person who brings him food says he hasn't opened the door for a month and the neighbors have heard him shouting.
On the doorstep there is a prostitute who doesn't move: to enter we have to squash ourselves against her breast.
We attack the climb methodically, there's not much air.
The stairway turns now right, now left,
outside it's getting dark and the few lightbulbs are burnt out.
The stairway smells of mold and cat piss.
Someone comes down with an electric torch, and we flatten ourselves against the wall so he can pass.
At every door a different smell: salt cod, pesto,
minestrone, couscous, chicken broth, we've skipped dinner.
At every door the music changes: melodic Neapolitan, Arab, reggae, techno, Genovese silence.

Having arrived, somehow, at the top of the stairs, we start the descent,
stopping to smell the flavors and listen to the noises,
to work out which is the door of our man:
we ring a few doorbells at random.
We wait to hear a shout, but Sergio is silent.

We are giving up hope, when a neighbor, through the small gap held closed by a chain, points at a door.
We ring, no noise, we knock.
Sergio is frail, old, he may not have eaten for days,
there are two of us, young and well-nourished,
so, once we are finally in,
and have entrusted the cat to the neighbor and closed the windows,
we have no trouble dragging him away with us.
We put him in the middle, I go ahead and Livio stays behind.

Going down is more difficult than coming up:
we can't see the steps and it would be easy to fall.
Every three steps an invective, an admonishment, a request for lights. Sergio stays silent.

Halfway down the stairs, the irreparable happens:
a gigantic guy is coming up, complete with guitar, and behind him another, both Senegalese, with a drum.
We are jammed like two lines of cars in a narrow street,
we deliberate in strange tongues,
begin to make strenuous and minuscule maneuvers, reverse, parallel, unbind, wriggle out,
the first passes but new ones appear:
it's an entire Senegalese band
with bass, keys, sax, backing singers.
When the stairs are clear again our bodies are battered and bruised.
But then comes a pregnant woman.
More careful moves and contortion gymnastics,
then we get down to the door.
Squeeze past the prostitute again.
We are outside: Livio and me. But where's the patient?

He's up there.
He's turned the lights back on and is waving at us from the window
his small hand against the sky.
We'll say we didn't find him.
It's easier to catch a macaque in a tree than a patient in the tall buildings of the back streets.

Chapter Five
Bad company

1.

Where did the drug addicts go, the pack of wolves that used to pound the alleys between Via Gramsci and Vico Untoria by night?
You would see them hunched over, fire in their eyes,
ears pricked up, nostrils flared.
They scratched at walls, examined doorways,
looked under cars, lifted pots of geraniums, brushed windowsills,
long fingers poking into every hole.
When you wander those streets now, they've all disappeared.
In which Siberia, under the light of which moon, does the hunt go on?

2.

Carmelo, you tell me you have stopped using.
But was it not you I saw yesterday rocking back and forth in the middle of Vico dei Macelli?
Was it not you forcing women with grocery bags to move out of the way to avoid collision?
It is true, you admit, it was me, but I had just had a drink.

Carmelo, someone who has had a drink staggers sideways, loses

their balance, takes two or three small steps to straighten up, then stops
and, if he doesn't crash into something, falls over.
The movements of someone who has had a drink are stilted.
You were rocking, standing still with your eyes half shut,
slowly leaning forward,
inch by inch, beyond normal limits
—now he's falling, he's falling—
but no,
you surpassed your center of gravity, like the tower of Pisa,
then returned vertical,
and immediately began to lean slowly again,
going down, down, headfirst,
so far you could pick a cigarette butt off the ground with your teeth.
Carmelo, someone who's had a drink doesn't rock like that.

3.

When you start out as a psychiatric consultant in the Emergency Room, gaining the trust of your colleagues is hard.
You are not only young but also a psychiatrist,
the interns and surgeons look down on you:
Sure, write up your consultation, but know that in here it's me who decides.

If the Emergency Room is unconquerable, there's always the waiting room,
the waiting room is behind the lines, somewhere you can infiltrate.
Look around to identify the psychiatric cases:
the one sitting in a corner still and silent, the one pacing around ranting, the one moving the chairs and the clock.

You can sit down and ask what the problem is, begin to resolve it.
If you can thin out the waiting room, word will travel fast:
a newfound respect amongst the doctors in the ER.

The waiting room is a world of its own, and it's already clinical:
there's a lot to learn.
There the aggressive are aggressive, the anxious are anxious,
that is reality, the medical examination is just a performance.

4.

They bring you into the ER, Carmelo: you have overdosed, already colder than hot.
Nurse Mara looks at you, then looks over to the doctor on the other side of the room
and moves her index finger to her elbow, the sign for intravenous.
The doctor nods yes.
Her hands move quickly, tick goes the plastic breaking, tack the vial snapping.
Mara bends over, searches with her finger, seeking from head to toe a vein, injects, stands up again.
You startle then breathe out: the opioid antagonist quickly kicks in.
Then your arms and legs begin to jerk around, each limb isolated like a marionette,
you open your eyes in amazement, lift your head. As soon as you see where you are, you snarl:
Bastard! You've taken my stuff away! Mind your own fucking business! Now I'm in withdrawal!
You get up and you leave, knocking into and insulting everyone in your path.

Three hours pass.

They bring you back, paler than before.
The doctor sees you and signals intravenous across the room to Mara.
Tick, tack, she bends, searches, injects.
You jolt, ignited:
you again, stupid bitch! You and all your kids go die! Shove the Narcan up your ass!
And you leave.
This time the nurse bursts into tears.

Three hours pass, the ambulance brings you back, you're deeper into your opioid coma,
but then you scream like a pig about to be slaughtered:
Bastards! I'm reporting you!
I, to salvage everyone's day and your skin, order a nice involuntary hospitalization: as I take you to Ward 77, the others reach over the stretcher with their fists clenched.

5.

A raving lunatic comes in, possibly drunk.
They open the doors to the ER to let him out without anyone getting hurt,
but he has no intention of leaving and trashes the place.
They call the on-shift psychiatrist, a phenomenon,
the kind of guy who wants to do everything himself.
With stealthy words he invites the giant to calm down, the latter hurls him against a stretcher, and the wretch scolds him vigorously. The brute launches himself forward, his two hands reaching for his neck.
And what does the wimp do?
He grabs tiny nurse Mara, by the shoulders,
as if she were a pillow with which to defend himself:

when the brute moves to the right, he shifts Mara to the right,
then brandishes her to the left,
at which point he looks around, sees the door, throws Mara onto the maniac and runs away.
Outside, all he can think to do is close the door behind him, shutting Mara in the room, alone, with the menace.
He even holds onto the handle, resisting the fists and shoulders trying to burst through, as she screams to the ceiling.

Mara sees me in the corridor today and whistles: you psychiatrists are worse than the drug addicts.
The surgeon walks away from me raising his scalpel: watch out, Milone.

6.

Will you stop asking passersby for money?
But why, doc, I'm offering them the chance to go to heaven for a few coins.

Carmelo, if God cares for such details, anyone who gives you a few coins for heroin
is going to hell.

7.

If two nurses are talking, nine times out of ten
they're talking about food:
what they ate yesterday,
what they'll eat tomorrow,
how their mamma used to cook,
their favorite food,

their nonna's special recipe,
what they ate at Christmas and New Year the last ten years,
what they'd like to eat at Christmas and New Year next year,
the thousand ways you can cook fungi and snails and osso buco,
the best restaurant in the city for meat, for fish, for coffee, for dessert.
The nurses at the old psychiatric hospital also spoke of nothing but food,
as do inmates in the darkness of their cells
and castaways at sea.

8.

Carmelo, you've been inside for six months and another six await you.
On one of my psychiatric visits, I come and see you in prison.
I go to the gym every day, you tell me,
and you extend a hand: want an arm wrestle?
Your cellmates gather round: come on!
We get set up and someone says: go!
I start at seventy percent ready to increase,
you push me down a little, eighty and I'm back up,
you push me down a little, ninety and I'm back up,
then we pause, precariously teetering, everyone watching and chanting: Carmelo! Carmelo!
You start to sweat, I give the little I have left
and slowly push you down.
I won! I leave radiant and set off on my Vespa.

At the first red light I stop and my mouth drops open:
I didn't let him win.
He is in prison for a year and I'm free, and I didn't let him win!
Cars are honking their horns behind me, but I don't move.

9.

You tell me that I have to prescribe you methadone and flunitrazepam in the doses you want,
because I am a public servant
and your taxes pay my salary.
Carmelo, I didn't know you paid income tax on what you pickpocket, mug, and burgle.

10.

Carmelo, when you are half done, you finish the job with words: on your feet rocking, eyes half-closed, you tell the world as you see it,
you listen to yourself, question yourself, respond to yourself,
you mumble, interrupt yourself, resume, sob,
hiccup,
one moment you are quiet, then impassioned, you protest, fart,
regurgitate, suspend the argument,
close your eyes, fall asleep,
you grumble, go quiet, grumble again, go silent,

there, you're done,
with words
the cheaper drug.

11.

Giulia, you ask me if drug addicts sometimes tell the truth.
Giulia, drug addicts are always lying, even when they're telling the truth.

12.

Emilio, you tell me that you take Viagra to visit prostitutes, you look at me and expect me to envy you,
then you tell me you take cocaine, and look at me and expect me to envy you,
then you tell me that you still masturbate, and look at me and expect me to envy you,
soon you'll tell me that you piss yourself and expect me to envy you.

13.

A white room.
In the entrance, blinding light: you have sold the curtains and the shutters.
We go into the other rooms, white, empty: you have sold the furniture, the pictures, the lighting fixtures.
A frail old woman moves around in the brightness, your mother.
It is obvious where she sleeps: in a corner, on an old dark blanket.
You have sold the beds and the bedside tables.
You have sold the fridge, the gas cooker, the TV, and the radio.
There is only one thing you haven't sold: the toilet. And your mother.
We mumble something about you, Carmelo.
You mother defends you: poor boy.

You walk back in with long strides,
you grunt, go into the bathroom, unscrew the toilet,
load it onto your shoulder, leave.

14.

Carmelo, how can a crime artist like you lower yourself to begging?
Things, with you, are never what they seem.
You hold out your hat but, at the same time, your cautious eyes are on the lookout, checking the movements of the police, giving hints to the bag-snatchers,
harvesting their loot, buying and selling small plastic bags.
Essentially, you are directing the traffic.

15.

Crying, you ask me to follow you assiduously as a doctor for the coming years.
Carmelo, your father, brothers, wife, and children have ditched you,
your friends, business partners, and your dog,
why on earth would I get involved?
Carmelo, even your creditors give you a wide berth,
why would I tether myself to you?

16.

Once upon a time, to recruit new nurses, head nurses from the mental asylums would knock on the doors of rural priests and round up the strapping men of the village.

Ferdinando, you were a farmer,
in the early years you treated the patients like donkeys and sacks of potatoes, the way you moved them around.
Everyone remembers the day when Andrea flew into a rage on

the ward, frightening everyone with his shouting and running up and down the corridors,
and with a single arm you lifted him,
like a kicking goat,
and, all the while talking about something else,
carried him under your arm as you worked: you had forgotten about him.

Now twenty years have passed and you've become a fine psychologist: when a new patient comes in,
your nose can predict what awaits.
I always arm myself with your judgment.

17.

You have gone teetotal and you criticize me for drinking too much wine: one glass a day.
But was it not you who used to gulp down three liters and then stumble around the old town from one dive bar to another?
I remember, even then you would scoff at my one glass.
Donato, you've changed all your habits bar one: breaking my balls.

18.

Donato, at the end of our lives, you and I will have drunk the same amount of wine,
just distributed differently.

19.

Syringes.

Mischievous syringes, already filled, hidden in a pocket,
waiting for the patient to turn around.
World champion syringes, filled in three seconds while the patient is fighting your colleague.
Heist syringes, injected through pants, through torn fishnet stockings.
Friendly fire syringes, stabbed into the hand of your colleague who is restraining the patient.
Masterful syringes, following the instructions to the letter while the patient looks on suspiciously.
Van Gogh syringes full of colorful solutions.
High-tech syringes of every density: liquid, flaky, oily, rubbery, tar.

Injections that numb, injections that wake.
The right injection in the wrong person, the wrong injection in the right person.
Injections left in the kitchen. Whose is this?
Bouncing, pounding, trembling, stabbing injections.

Listen, tiger: either you take the drops, or we'll have to give you an injection.
We'll have to give you an injection, tiger.
Tiger, are you going to let us do it or not?

20.

Ferdinando, a bit wild you have remained,
so, when you put on your white scrubs, it takes real effort to be gentle with the patients, but it is obvious that you would like to grab them by the neck the moment they threaten or disrespect you. You struggle against your nature and no patient or relative has ever come to complain,

you just need, once a day, to withdraw to the kitchen and curse to the ceiling:
Bastards, all bastards, pieces of shit, parasites,
it must be nice, not having to work every waking hour, gas the lot of them!
This suffices.
One final "bastards," then you plaster the smile back onto your face and return to the ward
to exercise your patience in order to earn your wages.

Yesterday an internist in a consultation meeting started to protest: But he's a Nazi. You have to get rid of him! Why aren't you getting rid of him?
Enrico, you do not know this, but he is one of the best nurses we have.

21.

Verdigris, so-called for the color of your skin,
but they could call you half moon
because you are thin and full of craters,
or Nosferatu for your long, black fingernails,
or knife for your razor-sharp nose,
or yellow fingers for the always-lit cigarette
held in the scornful corner of your mouth.
You pretend to be paralytic and go around in a wheelchair pushed by a bodyguard they say is armed.
You hate women, perhaps when you were young one rejected you, and now that you have the best heroin in the city and they are queueing up to satisfy your desires you can enjoy your revenge.
Why don't you at least wash a little?
The more disgusting you are, the more they are humiliated, the more you enjoy it.

22.

When we bring Carmelo in, he has to be frisked.
I witnessed this operation, carried out by a not-too-shrewd nurse:
the nurse makes him get undressed and checks his clothes;
in the meantime he, naked, holds up a little plastic bag and even gives me a wink,
I indicate the hand in the air to the nurse with my eyes.
Open your hand! he says, and passes the little bag into his other hand: it is so unfair that he has two hands!
Open both hands! But he coughs and brings one hand to his mouth.
Open your mouth! He opens it, but fixes his hair and places the bag on his head, holding it up by keeping his eyebrows raised.
And winks at me again.
Relax your forehead! the nurse orders.
He makes the little bag fall forward onto the floor and places a foot over it.

Let's stop now, I'll do it: I'm clocking off in half an hour.

23.

Rufo, on Ward 77 we look at your wedding photo on your desk,
we lightly brush your pens,
we move your umbrella, stroke your armchair, but you, where are you?
On the job you are perceived, mentioned, remembered, evoked, desired, called, invoked,
beseeched, begged,
but never seen.

Careful now, Giulia, let's repeat the lesson.
One patient swears he saw Rufo today standing at the foot of his bed: this is called a hallucination.
The patient who loves him swears she saw him flying around the kitchen: this is called a vision.
An Alzheimer's patient swears he talked to him a while ago: this is called confabulation.
A private patient phoned hoping to find him here: this is called delusion.
Giorgio the schizophrenic says that he is upstairs spying on us: this is called delirium.
I myself thought I saw him a moment ago in the corridor: this is called *déjà vu.*
Rufo, your absence looms large in our minds.
We live here like in Ithaca, waiting for Ulysses.

24.

Tito, you ask me to swap shifts with you:
Do it for me, I'm your friend.
If I ask you to swap shifts with me, you tell me:
Don't ask me, I'm your friend.
Tito, I pay double for your friendship, while you pay nothing.

25.

Marcello, when a patient comes in who speaks of himself with acronyms:
I have OCD and PD treated at the PCC with TCA and BDZ, there's nothing you can do.

26.

Why do I like living by the sea?
Inland the assholes are 360 degrees around you.
By the sea they're only 180. The rest is water.

27.

Overdose is a train that zooms by in the night.
Carmelo, when you passed through
I didn't see you at the window.
The next day you simply weren't here.
I remember your quick glance,
your deeply inhaled cigarette,
your pointed shoes.

I don't remember a word, a thought, a feeling:
nothing of what you said to me was true.
Finally, nobody accompanied you to the station, nobody helped you to carry your baggage.
Everything remained still, as your train entered the tunnel.

28.

How will the next wave be?
Higher, more impetuous than the last?
And you wager, wait for it, watch it.
All the same, all different.
This game can keep going forever,
the great metronome never tires.
But for me, to leave, it is enough to have forgotten why I came.

29.

My cousin has a bit of anxiety, what can he take?
My cousin takes Ativan, is that O.K.?
My cousin doesn't sleep at night, what can he do?
Riccardo, I can't treat you through a middleman.
We've given your cousin, over the years, a wife, children, a job, debts, illnesses
and even a lover, to justify his anxieties,
but this cousin doesn't exist.
I'm fed up of treating the cousins of surgeons.

30.

Lino, thin as a beanstalk, tattooed like a fresco, you have few teeth left but cunning still twinkles deep in your eyes.
You have made peace with yourself,
you move lightly like a ghost, quietly, observing,
but you were a heavy addict in the past,
lord of the alleyways, king of heroin,
hellion of jail and the psych ward.
You survived drugs, fights, and even madness.
You escaped the slaughter of AIDS:
saved a thousand times by the doctors of infectious diseases
—soldiers in the trenches for years—
not one of them retreated and in the end they won.

Lino, now that you spend your days stroking cats
and there is almost wisdom in your eyes,
now that the volcano has burnt itself out, tell me:
what was the meaning of all this? What have you learned?
What do you have to say about the world,
you, who have lived so convulsively

and now tread the earth with such light footsteps.

31.

I have just finished restraining a 220-pound aggressive drunk
when the ER doctor appears:
There's another patient to see,
and nods toward the room next door.
I make a mistake here: instead of recomposing myself,
still sweaty, red-eyed and breathing heavily, I enter.
You, who have just heard the shouting, the abuse, the moving beds and thumps against the walls,
look at me with terror and take refuge on the far side of the room.

Our first encounter, Ines.
But this is the beautiful thing about our job:
You go from wrestling a bull
to extending a hand for a fluttering butterfly to land.

32.

Ward 77 is a locked ward.
When a new doctor arrives, a bunch of keys is thrust in his face and he is told: this is power.
I too, when I received the keys, swore to respect the rules:
when I open a door, I must remember to close it behind me, always,
I must not leave the keys lying around on tables and desks,
I must not leave the keys in the door,
cardinal sin,
I must not lose the keys, dishonor and sneering,

I must not forget the keys at home,
I must not lend the keys to anybody.

I am always distracted and slipping up, so, two or three times a day, the patients bring me the keys that I've left somewhere or other: Take them, doctor, they whisper,
so that my colleagues won't hear and admonish me.

33.

Whatever tension you feel during the workday,
the small weight of the keys calms you down.
You pass time stroking the pocket where the keys lie. When you cannot feel that weight, you worry,
not because you feel trapped, but because your colleagues will make you wait ten minutes to open any door.

I get the keys out, I open the door. I take a step, I close it behind me: I have forgotten something.
I get the keys out again, open the door again. I take a step, close it behind me: I get what I forgot.
I get the keys out again, open the door again. I take a step, close it behind me: the telephone rings in the room.
I get the keys out again . . . this is my day.
I dream of a Ward 77 with no keys, or at least with automatic doors.
In the meantime patients tell me: you're lucky you have keys.
Yes, I have the keys, but I am always here.

34.

Your father came in drunk to the Emergency Room, Lucrezia,

he screamed at me that it's my fault you killed yourself
and he swore to me, his hands in fists,
that sooner or later he'd make me pay.

Your mother came in crying,
she thanked me for everything I did for you,
she was almost caressing me,
she told me that she'd never be able to repay me.
Then she opened a tin box and showed me a little lead soldier on horseback, an old watch of mine, a pair of glasses I never spent long looking for, and an entire bunch of keys to the ward: fifteen keys.
She said: they were in Lucrezia's wardrobe.
Doctor, are they yours?

I have never seen them, ma'am. They are Lucrezia's.

35.

Keys are for locking the madness into Ward 77 when you go home.

36.

Now it is no longer you phoning me, Lucrezia,
but I wake up all the same.
Your father is right.
Why did I take you off lithium two months ago?
Nobody knows.
You had been asking for six months, but why did I do it?
Nobody knows. Except for you and me.

37.

The last time I saw you on the ward,
did you already know what you were going to do?
Did you come in especially to say goodbye?
And did I say goodbye when you left? I don't remember.
I hope I said goodbye.

Yes, I said goodbye: I raised my hand.
But why in that moment did I have the most fleeting of feelings
that it might be the last time?
Is that what happened?
If that's what happened,
why didn't I catch you up, stop you, talk to you?

If I wake myself up one more time, I'll lose my mind.

Chapter Six
If you were not you, if I were not me

1.

Who are you disturbing the dust on my doormat
for the first time
and stepping cautiously into the wisteria room?
Who are you sweeping your gaze over my books?
Who are you sighing as you sit down on my armchair and then
look up at my face through your eyelashes?
I know only that your name is Chiara.

2.

In the doorway my eyes, without my volition, asked: who are you?
Yours, without your volition, indicated the rain on the glass.
Then we introduced ourselves to each other with appropriate words for the occasion.
They weren't necessary.
We were already intimate, your sadness and me.

3.

Chiara, you are like a little plant in a vase.

You are separated, you live with two small children:
if no man waters you with a bit of attention,
you become dry, your head bowed and leaves falling
—even if you try to beat your feathers—
but if it is cloudy, just a drop is enough,
a passing compliment,
as umbrellas are opened in the wind,
and you lift your head
your petals unfurl
you let your leaves breathe
and you come to me with clear eyes,
anxious to know
if the world is still beautiful.

4.

You have come to me because you don't want the sadness to distract you,
you have to raise two children,
you don't want them to see you sick.
I believe it and I tell you: you can do it.
It will just take a bit more effort.

5.

The day passes from one duty to another
for the women who arrive breathless in the wisteria room.

The buzzer of the factory rings,
the bell of the convent rings,
the siren of the prison rings.

I too gave up the idea of freedom many years ago.
But for some time now the air has felt lighter,
dogs bark,
there is movement around and the evening sunset is serene,
the light persists:
perhaps it is too early to say, perhaps I am wrong,
but I feel that the sentence is about to end.
From one moment to the next, I expect to hear the screech of the bolt sliding.

6.

It is daytime and I am at the hospital.
Nighttime and I am at the hospital.
Raining and I am at the hospital.
Snowing and I am at the hospital.
The sun is shining and I am at the hospital.
Outside there is nobody, they're all at the beach
and I am at the hospital.
Outside there is an eerie sense of anticipation and I am at the hospital.
Outside there is the G8 and I am at the hospital.
Outside they are shooting and I am at the hospital.
The city is burning and I am at the hospital.
An atomic bomb has gone off in the port and I am at the hospital.
Aliens are coming down on long cables over Carignano and I am at the hospital.
The Horsemen of the Apocalypse gallop by outside with sharpened swords and I am at the hospital.
Outside Judgment Day is over, God is clearing out, the final lights of the Universe are dimmed,
and I am at the hospital.

•

7.

It's still me, I've just shaved my beard this morning!
I have not substituted Milone during the night, I haven't killed him and eaten him.
Filippo, it's me.
It'll take me twenty days to regrow my beard, how am I supposed to work now?

8.

And while I am here going up and down these hospital stairs,
in atonement for an inscrutable crime,
I hear sirens ring out:
the boats are leaving the port for South America,
the boats are leaving the port for Africa.

9.

You tell me that for you happiness is narrow,
sadness has a thousand rooms,
happiness is sterile, sadness fertile,
happiness is vulgar, sadness noble,
happiness is sad, sadness comforting,
happiness is foolish, sadness wise,
happiness is fleeting, sadness loyal.
You stop and look at me: you are worried that I don't understand.
Chiara, I could multiply your list by a thousand.

10.

It skips from cobble to cobble down the hill,
comes out on Corso Firenze and spreads
in the Spianata Castelletto, pooling into a lake, almost.
It is sucked down the steep descent toward the Meridiana piazza,
tumultuous, dragging every rolling object with it,
gushing through the old town,
bouncing down the marble steps of the little square,
swirling around itself, undecided,
then drops fast onto Via Quattro Canti
between the closed shutters and lost-looking dogs,
it is joined by the water that comes from other alleyways and streams and bursts from manholes
and crashes out of gutters and drainpipes,
runs unstoppable down Via Posta Vecchia, funneled through the Loggia di Banchi, mirroring San Pietro church
and finally emerging into the vastness of Piazza Caricamento,
here it spreads and softens, slow as destiny, up to the edges of the large stone square and, in a feeble cascade,
tumbles into the immense bowl of the port,
where it becomes calm, melting
and joins with those of a million years before.

The sea carries all the tears in the world.

11.

Filippo, you are convinced that the world is about to end.
You have sorted everything out and you look at me with a sadness that says: I'm sorry we're going to die.

Filippo, I'm here thinking about my stomach and how cold my feet are.
We are full of terrible thoughts.

12.

If you know someone, you have a duty toward them.
Better to not know anyone.

13.

Andrea, you are naked and immobile, defenseless,
ridiculed at work, ridiculed by the others,
to put food on the table for your family.
Where has your self-respect gone?
And your decency, tenderness, and pain?
It lies in subterranean pools, to which no one knows the path,
where some evenings, sure that you're alone,
you tiptoe down to bathe
with slow and silent movements.

I will not try to find your secret pathways,
I will not try to see how your relationship with yourself is reborn,
but how I would love to know the sacred source
from which flows the water that spreads
and blesses the forest and the mountain
and the sky, and each one of us.

14.

You cross your legs with the naturalness of the wind
ruffling your hair.
I will say nothing of your smile,
of your dark eyes,
or of how, sometimes,
you lightly arch your back to infinity.
Look but don't touch, Chiara. I know.
And so why at the end of the session
is my hair ruffled,
as if your hand has run through it.

15.

You sit down and your body goes with you,
seated in the middle of the room,
impatiently waiting for us to finish speaking.
You unconsciously hold your body the furthest away from me
you can: so that it won't distract me.
I too can feel my body. It is fidgeting.
We go on talking, indifferent, as if your body and mine don't exist.

But your body is a white horse in the middle of the room, and
mine is a black horse.
Noli me tangere. But horses don't know Latin.

16.

I go slowly through the gate on my Vespa and enter the large
tree-covered park, I am in the most beautiful neighborhood of
the city, a stone's throw from the sea.

In front of me: pavilions, courtyard gardens, raised passages.
I go inside to get the keys for the service car: marble floors, infinite rooms, higher than high ceilings, glass, light.
Each time I walk on these lawns, I touch these walls, I think: I would like to live here.
Then I check myself: it's the former Quarto asylum!

Here it is, the old white Panda. There is chewing gum on the seat, I get in, put the key in holding my breath: the engine starts up straight away. It's small, uncomfortable, the rubbery steering wheel, the hard clutch, but it moves. I'm coming to get you, Filippo.
The journey begins, Vittorio and I are taking you to the Community.

17.

Filippo, you need confines more than oxygen,
because identity is a confine.
And so I, an anarchist by nature, am forced to build walls.
First inside you, like walls in a house. Then outside and around you.
And they are thick walls, good high ones.
The freedom to knock them down, we'll sort that later.

18.

Shall we go back and pick him up again? I say.
I was thinking the same, admits Vittorio.
We have left Filippo in a Community in the mountains, hidden among chestnut trees and pines.
We left in the Panda five minutes ago, and we are already having second thoughts.

It would take me four days to go crazy in a place like that.
Two days for me.
What shall we do?
We hope that Filippo will get angry and break everything, so that we can admit him to Ward 77. Then we can hide him away.

19.

Are there indicators for fear of death? Of course. The simplest one is our average daily mileage.
Calculated by dividing the miles we travel in a year, car, train, plane included, by 365.
Mine is 50 miles a day.
Rufo, with all the conferences he attends, exceeds 300 miles a day.
As we know, death starts following us when we are born and walks behind us our whole life,
until one day she catches up and touches a shoulder. Lightly.

Now, if someone puts so many miles a day between himself and death, it means he is pretty damn fearful.
But the pursuer is a methodic and untiring walker.
She'll always bridge the distance.

20.

When my mother used to be late coming home, my father would mumble: Maria's probably found a funeral.
She was made that way: couldn't resist a funeral.
I must have got that from her.
When I come across a funeral, I feel the muscles in my legs pulling me toward it, I feel tears coming to my eyes and comforting words to my lips,

and I have to force myself to stick to my original route.

21.

You can see that you have not yet noticed yourself.
You have not yet noticed that you are alive,
in this limited place we call Earth,
for a limited time we call life,
within a limited confine we call body,
with a limited property we call I.
But you can't be woken up with a snap of the fingers.

Anyway, Filippo, what does it matter?
Nobody ever notices.

22.

Filippo, you who have succeeded in passing through,
and now are all scratches, sweat, dirt, tell me what it's like on the other side.
There where there is no reason.
I pore over large maps of the border.
By which hidden trails, which crossings, gullies, crags, did you manage to pass?
Tell me what it's like.

23.

Anna, at breakfast you open the fridge and shout: there's no milk!
I then go to the hospital and I can't manage to understand the people who want to kill themselves,

because I am so unsettled by your anger that I forgot to buy milk.

24.

Gloria, today in our session you are embarrassed, you hint, you allude, you imply that you are falling in love with me.
Delicate situation: when we talk about certain things we make only trouble.
I cannot reject your affection so as not to humiliate you,
I cannot appreciate it so as not to mislead you,
I cannot ignore it so as not to disregard you.
I am stuck.
You are the first to downplay it, saying:
It is inevitable, it happens: it is positive transference.

Culture! Giving a name to things kills them. And so it is.
A strange sadness hangs in the air.
Along with many of my worries.

25.

Three years have passed and I still feel your absence, Lucrezia.
Every time I am in trouble,
and a thousand screeching reasons pull me in different directions,
I look around in vain for your clear eyes.

26.

Anna, a mosquito bites you in bed,

you make so much noise that you wake the neighbors' dog,
who wakes all the dogs on the block.
The power of a mosquito: it has woken a neighborhood.

27.

Chiara, you feel lonely.
It is August, the whole valley is in love.
Closing your eyes, holding your nose, blocking your ears doesn't help. The summer is blinding.
You don't know where to go.
The world's lust for life is killing you.

28.

Depressives use the past tense:
I made a mistake, I didn't manage . . .
or the present but with a deep link to the past:
I am to blame, I am a failure.
Euphorics use the imperative: come, do, buy
and the future: we'll celebrate, we'll conquer, we'll meet.
Schizophrenics get it all wrong: they say I am instead of I was, I will be, I would be, if I were.
People with personality disorders, always the imperative: write, give me, listen to me, obey.
Neurotics are charming people who use the conditional: could I, would you be so kind . . .
or the second conditional: if it were possible, if you were sure it wouldn't be a bother . . .
Giulia, be wary of people who use the third conditional: if I had been, if I had had. They're the worst.

29.

At each of life's disappointments you withdraw to your secret garden, built over years of pain and care.
Life is ugly, your garden has a thousand roses: there is an orchard you seeded the year your husband left you,
there is a garden of herbs cultivated the spring you lost your job and there is a lemon tree planted when your sister passed, out of season, but it's grown well anyway.

You have never said a word to anyone about your secret garden. Not even to me. But it is there that you go when you are not listening to me.
I am sure: I can smell it.
How I would like to come and see it, Chiara. And indeed I come closer, but you keep me outside the gate, throwing rocks at me.

30.

Inside you there is a sky full of clouds even if it's sunny outside.
I remember that it rained like that on my mother's face: it rained, it rained and the water came up to the gateway.
But Papà, looking at his barometers, just said: it's not raining.

Now I am no longer afraid of the great flood and I am calm sitting here, while inside you the rain has been pouring down for days.
Hail today.
You have lost the middle seasons, Chiara: it's fire or ice.

31.

I visit Filippo in the Therapeutic Community three months after he went in.
This time I take the highway, then get lost in the forest and wind back and forth over one mountain then the other.
Filippo is happy to see me, he seems more robust, his cheeks are red and his hands are calloused.

I look at him and look around. And I wonder:
For what is Filippo rehabilitating here? What can he learn?
He can learn to distinguish a swallowtail from a white admiral.
To distinguish the behaviors of black ants from red ants.
To distinguish a northerly wind from a southwesterly.
To distinguish Sirius from Aldebaran.

And in the long winter?
He can learn to distinguish the seven types of snow.
He can study the tracks of wild boar, hares, and foxes.
He can learn to make granita from icicles and lemon.

All splendid, and useful in life if he later becomes a hunter in Montana, but of course other things risk being unlearnt.
Like how to go into a store and buy bread.
How to use the elevator.
How to say hello to someone in the street.

Filippo, when he is discharged and goes back to the city,
the first time he crosses the road,
will forget to look both ways.

32.

Psychiatry is eighty percent an ethical profession.
And twenty percent plain old hard work.

33.

I come with you and open the door
to see you out.
You already have one foot on the threshold,
when you turn to say goodbye.

I take in every last scent of you
because winter is coming.

You leave.

34.

If you were not ill . . .
If you were not bipolar . . .
If I were not your doctor . . .
If I had met you, in a store, in the street, at the beach, in another world . . .
maybe . . .

Chiara, if you were not you and I were not me.

35.

My wife saw it before I did.

Paolo, why on Wednesdays do you change your shoes and shirt and spruce yourself up?

36.

After many interviews in the wisteria room
you are admitted to Ward 77 for a treatment adjustment, you are running a high fever,
and I am supposed to tell you: get undressed, I need to examine you.
I hide in the kitchen like a burglar and wait for a colleague to come in.
When he does I tell him:
you touch her.

37.

You secretly came looking for me,
you wanted to see where I lived,
what the street I walk down every day is like,
what my eyes see from the window.
And, most importantly, if the flowers in my garden are well looked after.
You had prepared a good excuse, in case you bumped into me.

Maybe you were hoping to bump into me, you wanted me to know, without having to tell me.
Maybe you were afraid of bumping into me: you weren't sure what color your cheeks would go.
Maybe you were even more afraid of not bumping into me, you'd have been disappointed.

Maybe, you didn't even come.

38.

There, those are Chiara's footsteps: she's coming down the stairs, I look at myself in the mirror, fix my hair,
polish the points of my shoes on my pant leg.
I never do that.

39.

The first time it happens to you, you are shocked:
have I fallen in love with a patient?
I think about her, I like her, I desire her . . .

If I have fallen in love it's a problem: I am more interested in having her than in curing her. But what does it matter: if we love each other, love will cure all her wounds. But is that really how it works? I should abandon her as a doctor and pursue her as a man, but if I leave her as a patient, will we still be in love with each other? Maybe we'll look at each other and ask: who are you?

Now not only am I in love and full of desire, but I'm becoming a fool.

40.

But does she notice my embarrassment?
Of course she does.
She is a war machine who understands everything in two ways:
One because she's sick, the other because she's a woman.

She sits down in front of me and one buttock moves on the chair, she moves a cheek, raises her eyebrow: she is moving too much!
My heart and my breath accelerate.
Why does she pretend it's nothing?

41.

Lucky psychoanalysts who get to hide behind the patient.
They can go red, cry, yawn,
and even, if they want, sleep.
We battle in full daylight.

If get to be reborn, I'll be a psychoanalyst.

42.

I accompanied you to the exit and opened the door of the office.
You stopped in the doorway facing the open world.
Too much light flooded your eyes.
Too much noise invaded your ears.
Too much heat hit your skin.
You leaned for a moment backward, toward the shade and the silence.
You smiled at me again. *We can't. We can't.*
You leaned forward again.
You left.

43.

If I treat you with unkindness, you cry:

this is what I've always got from life.
If I treat you with kindness, you cry:
this is what I've never got from life.
Tina, you cry either way.

44.

I treat as many patients as I can,
So that I don't become too fond of any of them.

45.

Wake up!
But you don't move a muscle.

Don't wake me up until there is snow outside.
Don't wake me up until the cold is freezing the trees.
Don't wake me up until the wolf is following the scent of the lamb.
Don't wake me up until the vulture is tracing circles in the sky.
Don't wake me up until justice is so difficult it is renounced.
Don't wake me up until the truth reveals itself.

I place my hand on your shoulder and repeat: wake up.
You don't move a muscle.
Your time is still to come.

46.

Marcello, when they call you into the Emergency Room,

stand outside the patient's room
and listen.

Absolute silence: a depressive.
Depressives do not make any sound with their hands and feet, they hold their breath, occasionally crying softly.
It could be a neurotic, but only time will tell:
sooner or later a neurotic will let some sound out.

Continuous sounds, the most varied: footsteps, doors and windows being slammed, open and then closed,
chairs moved and then put back into place: it's a euphoric.
Euphorics are always handling the world, but in trying to make it better they sabotage it.
However it could also be someone who's intoxicated with cocaine or other psychostimulants.

Nonstop crying, sobbing, scraping of chairs, moaning:
it's not a depressive, it's a hysteric.
Accelerated breathing and gasping: a crisis of anxiety
—sorry: a panic attack.

Identifying a schizophrenic is more difficult,
but a rhythmically repeated clicking sound,
a strange grumbling, exaggerated rasping, loud flatulence, and an unrelenting lullaby
can be sufficient.

Then there are the sad sounds:
continuous incomprehensible whining with sporadic shouting can be the calling card for a patient with severe dementia or mental disabilities.

47.

Bianca, for months you have been circling a black cloud, hinting, stopping, turning around, looking at me,
you would like me to understand by myself, but I don't understand.
Today I understood: once a week, in the afternoon, you visit a man and let yourself be beaten for as long as he wants.
Sometimes it takes a while.

When we are talking about it, if I raise my voice or use the wrong word you cry,
I try to be as gentle as possible,
but I always get it wrong, my tone or the way I look or the way I breathe
and you end up crying.
I, who would never hit you, always make you cry.

48.

The sea is like your dog.
If you get close, it licks you and jumps up at your legs.
Then it starts playing, going back and forth,
skipping here and there.
If you throw a piece of wood it retrieves it.
When you start walking away, it keeps wagging its tail
and whimpering for you to come back.
Try feeling alone, with a sea like that.

49.

She's back again, of her own accord,
she arrived without warning, without phoning.

Once again she came into the house with her boots covered in mud.
She looked around full of scorn
and sat down at the head of the table legs spread wide,
she banged on the counter with her fists and ordered you to bring her something to eat.
I guess the Porsche will stay parked where it is for a while.
Your second mistress has returned, Emilio: sadness.

50.

Lucrezia, today in the ER I met a young girl of twenty
who had your same crafty smile.
She was shouting and smashing everything
while I, lucky me, enjoyed watching.
Calm down, my dear! slipped out, so affectionate she stopped for a moment to study me, as surprised as the nurses around us.
Everyone stood still for three seconds. Then the bedlam began again.
She was you.

I admitted her and looked after her,
but as I was about to write on her chart, I stopped myself.
And asked Tito to take care of it.

51.

Chiara, now you look at me calmly and say:
Doctor, I'm embarrassed to say it, but at this point between us . . .
There was a period that I found myself thinking: is he interested in me? Yes, he's interested.

Then, after a while: but is he interested?
There were times when your cheeks flushed and I would think to myself: See, he is interested.

It's a good job that we never talked about it, that we didn't ruin everything.
Together, we have created something.

52.

By this point I know everything about you, Chiara.
You have told me about your mother's death, your father's illness, about when you were molested at the cinema as a little girl and when you were abused, I know about your husband's betrayals, your fears for your children, I know about the tensions with your office manager and your secret loves.
I know everything about you, Chiara.
But I don't know what biscuits you eat in the morning or how you brush your teeth, I don't know if you snore at night or if you move around in your sleep, I don't know what your breath smells like or how you rub your feet,
I don't know what you say when you make love or how you bite your tongue,
I don't know how you walk in the rain,
how you stroke your cats,
I don't know the look in your eyes when you gaze out of the window.
Chiara, about you I know only the unimportant things.

53.

Wake me up, before you leave.

Don't let me be woken by the sound of the door closing behind you.
By the sounds of your footsteps as you descend the stairs
and the bang of the front door as it closes onto the street.

54.

I know that I'll never see you again.
And I have to say it's for the best.

Chapter Seven
The Lady

1.

Miriam, unknown person, it's your first time in hospital.
You enter Ward 77, you take five steps,
you open a door at random,
a nurse is talking on the phone, the window is wide open,
you throw yourself out.
All within ten seconds. Entrance and exit.
The nurse's mouth is still open.
Who were you, Miriam?

2.

Why did she do it? your mother asks me.
I smile in a way that says everything and nothing.
At least she's no longer suffering, she says,
then she looks at me with narrowed, searching eyes:
that's why she did it, isn't it?
I smile in a way that says yes and no.
Neither of us consoled, we go our separate ways.
Now that I'm alone, I ask you, Lucrezia:
why did you do it?

3.

Once when I was young, an older psychiatrist told me that very few people kill themselves by choice.
I smiled at him, but inside I was thinking:
oh come on! I don't believe that.
He, having read my mind, added: in time you'll understand.

4.

You jumped from the fourth floor, Elia.
It must have been luck, your sixteen years, the hand of God: death was eluded.
Now you look up at me from your bed in intensive care, lifting your big eyes from your ten broken bones,
and you ask me, with sincere astonishment: who pushed me?
Elia, there is no doubt, you pushed yourself.
But you have never had problems, you were getting ready for school like any other day.
Who pushed me? you ask again.
It will take us some years now, Elia, you and I, to find out who pushed you.

5.

I want you to call me immediately for every non-fatal suicide by jumping.
The head nurse in ER looks at me perplexed:
you mean the survivors?
Yes.
Even in the night?
Yes.

Even on your days off?
Yes.
Even if they don't speak?
Yes. I want to see them as soon as they arrive, but, please, only ones who have jumped from the third floor or higher.
Why from the third floor or higher?
To be sure they were intending to die.
Why's that?
I have a suspicion that they do not jump voluntarily.
What are you talking about! Don't wind me up.
Think about it for a moment.
Milone, provided you, and this will mean going against your nature, stand still and silent in a corner, and don't make a fuss, don't touch anything . . .
then maybe . . .
Deal.

6.

Oh, the autumn of that year!
There was a wind over Genoa,
a wind so strong that people rose up and fell down one by one,
from this sloping city, full of steps, high walls,
windows onto the sky.
And that wind still blew in the spring and the following autumn and the next year still.

A shoe still lies on a windowsill,
a cigarette butt at the foot of a balustrade,
a pair of glasses on a balcony.

7.

I have begun a game of hide-and-seek with the Lady,
but I must be careful: death is touchy,
a click of the fingers and she'll make me my own hit man.
The perfect crime.

8.

I've known you for years, Ludovica, when one morning you are brought into the ER. She jumped from the fifth floor, they say on the phone, do you want to come?
I run. There are six of them around you, they are finishing cutting your clothes off with scissors. There's the surgeon, the resuscitator, and four nurses grappling with wires and tubes.
It's like a wall, I can't get though.
Milone, don't get in the way, let us work. Come back tomorrow if you want to mess around.
She'll be on drugs tomorrow,
the pages of the book will be closed,
I want to talk to her now
and I push until the youngest nurse makes an opening for me.
You want to see the show, Milone? the surgeon says. Here it is.
I keep my eyes open but I would like to close them.
It's a miracle, she's alive. She must have twenty broken bones, now we're looking at her internal organs.
You are a swollen sack, black, unrecognizable,
but, incredibly, you are conscious and you recognize me!
Doctor, what happened? you whisper with great effort.
You jumped from the fifth floor, Ludovica.
No, it's not possible. Don't believe them, Doctor . . .
There were five witnesses, a nearby policeman clarifies.

I let myself fall back into a chair.
Milone, the surgeon says, can't you handle a failed suicide?
No, I can't handle what they say.

9.

A person does not attempt suicide due to a quantitively larger suffering—suicide happens in a qualitatively different state of mind.
No imagination or experience of living people can help us understand it.

10.

Lucrezia, would you also have said: I didn't want to die?
Maybe it wasn't that you acted, but just stopped resisting.
In your own way, you made the decision.

11.

Thinking of suicide as a voluntary act serves only to reassure ourselves: if I don't want to, I won't do it.
But is that really true?

12.

Why am I so interested in suicide?
After ten years, I heard the breath of the enormous black bat in the darkness.
And the question: boy, are you sure you want to keep going?

I retreated from the study of suicide.

13.

I say it in a low voice, so that the Lady doesn't hear me:
In fact, in this job we are always working on suicide.

14.

In the dictionary it says: suicide is a voluntary act.
The philosophers say: suicide is an extreme expression of human freedom.
I am a psychiatrist, not a philosopher:
you'll never hear me calling it voluntary.
For many clinical psychiatrists, suicide is the extreme proof of humans' lack of freedom.

15.

A smart-ass asks me to admit him, he threatens suicide. Then, seeing my puzzlement, bitter and offended he observes: what do you know about pain!
You won't commit suicide, I say. You don't have what it takes.
How dare you! If I kill myself you'll be taken to court.
As far as I'm concerned, you're discharged.
Let me speak with the head physician! I want another psychiatrist!

16.

Livia, you go around saying you're going to kill yourself in one year and you've set the date, time, and method.
I am happy: for a year I can relax.

17.

Lisetta, you are angry that I don't say the things you want,
at the time you want,
in the tone of voice you want,
with the intention you want
and the thoughts you want.
Lisetta, it is not exactly easy.

18.

In many cases, saying that suicide is a choice
adds insult to injury.

19.

They arrive in the Emergency Room together like a bolt of lightning in a cloudless night.
She, Pinuccia, asks me to admit her anorexic daughter.
Her daughter, Giorgina, two eyes on a little pile of bones, refuses and laughs in my face.
She, Pinuccia, insists and threatens me, as if this were the first and last chance of treatment: if you don't admit my daughter, I'll report you to the judiciary.
Signora Pinuccia, after fifteen years of quietly waiting,

did you need to decide,
right at midnight on my Christmas shift,
to force your daughter into treatment?

Giorgina shouts: if you admit me I'll kill myself!
In response, her mother shouts: if you don't admit her I'll report you!

Ladies, calm down, it's Christmas Eve.
The best thing would be for you to go home and continue your usual routines. Then, if you want to, you can come back and make this scene again at midnight on New Year's Eve.
But do book your tickets, because that night there's usually a line of people who want to change their lives.

20.

If one veil is lifted from the question of suicide
another appears in its place.
Suicide is made up of endless labyrinths and tricks,
every attempted suicide is different.
Like a mirage, the closer you get to it, the further away it becomes.

21.

Marcello, it is indecent to talk about death, but murder is a topic that's encouraged in society. It relaxes, reassures.
It gives the illusion that it is we who control death.
Once the murderer is arrested, nobody else dies.
Everybody safe at home.

22.

But it is not true that a murderer has control over death.
Just like those who attempt suicide, murderers decide nothing.

23.

Sad people leave the house less and spend less than happy people.
The ideal for consumerist society is that everybody's happy and no one is sad.
Sadness is a subversive mental state.

24.

Consumerist society has nothing to say about death
for the simple fact that dead people do not consume.

25.

With Giorgio we have a gentlemen's agreement.
When he feels the impulse to kill himself, he lets us know and asks to be restrained.
There's no joking with him, he is capable of taking a run-up and ploughing headfirst into the wall.
We carry out our side.
After half an hour, when he's better, he asks to be unbound.
We do it.
We are calm, we leave him alone, he's not thinking about suicide anymore.

Many people are dead because of half an hour. Some because of much less.
It's called a suicidal crisis. It comes and goes.

26.

If the person who commits suicide is not to blame,
how can the people who love them be?

27.

Livia, do you remember?
Every morning for months you dragged yourself out on a walk.
The dogs and cats in the street recognized your footsteps, and the lizards on the walls,
and the caretaker at the gate with the broom in his hand.
You would stop at the burial recess you had bought in the shade of the tallest cypress, you would stand there, undecided whether to throw yourself into the tomb, as was your right.
You forced yourself to leave again only because your children were waiting at home. On the way home you would stop a hundred times to look back, sighing.
Do you remember?

You chose, after a month of trying on, your death dress,
the white lacy one,
you laid it out on the seat next to the bed
and smoothed out the little pleats every evening,
then you went to say goodbye to your friends, myself included.
Do you remember?
As soon as I saw you coming in, I wrote you a prescription for antidepressants.

*

Livia, how can you say that you no longer want to take them because you've put on a few pounds!

28.

You are scared that the medicines will take possession of your mind and therefore you refuse them.
You are wrong, Livia: it is the depression that takes possession of your mind, the medicine gives the key back to its rightful owner.

29.

Adriano, you say that depression brings you closer to suicide, but that your will is important:
it is the man who gives or withholds his consent to leave.
Like the farmer gives or withholds his consent to the river, when he sees it rising and submerging his fields, his animals, his house, himself.

Many victims of suicide are silent bystanders.

30.

It is often said that you kill yourself in a moment of lucidity.
Wouldn't it be better to say that you save yourself in a moment of lucidity?
Strange that lucidity would kill you.

31.

One of the many tricks of the suicidal person:
some who kill themselves, seen or heard an hour earlier,
were not in fact depressed.
It can happen that a depression, even a serious one, can come over you in minutes.
You are whistling when you start shaving your beard, and as you rinse the razor you are looking around
wondering how to end it.

The unpredictability is what's scary, we can't even conceive of it. Better to think that it is we who control suicide.

32.

Lino, you have been in hospital for ten days, closely observed by several doctors and nurses,
I am there too,
but you seem so calm,
one evening you ask to go out into the corridor for a walk.
You go up to the top floor, you take flight.

Knowing that a person is at the point of suicide is difficult,
even for a group of specialists.
Nobody can expect that of themselves.

Fortunately, the opposite also happens:
sometimes, in the ER or the clinic,
we talk with a patient
and, without even realizing, we save him from suicide.
He'll tell us himself, years later, when we meet on the street
and he thanks us

and we think,
Who is this guy? What did I do for him?

33.

Lorenzo, you called me into the ER because two patients were fighting and bothering the nurses.
I came all the way there for a pair of thugs.
The same day, a gentleman who had been sitting patiently for three hours in your waiting room, not uttering a word, got up and threw himself off the high wall in front of the hospital.
Lorenzo, do not call me for the patients who raise their voices, call me for the ones who are silent.

34.

I was overwhelmed by sadness after today's rostering meeting.
Rufo, it is not because you used all the tricks in the book,
it is not because you lied.
It is because we have worked together for fifteen years,
and we will continue to work together,
and I can't get my head around how you can be willing to forgo my respect, trust, and friendship, to get yourself, through pure duplicity,
two afternoons and two nights.
And I wonder, if this is how you treat me, your colleague who you see every day, how do you treat the patients who come into the ER, who you meet only once in your life?

35.

My patients work alongside me,
the ones who wield the final blow are my colleagues.

36.

Franca, a young doctor in the Emergency Room,
you have the lively, attentive eyes of one who has not worked here long.
The waiting room is full to the brim, the nurses are angry.
Shouts, noises, movements, shoves,
how long will it take for you to become cynical?
In Genoa there is a saying: "he's drunk the water of the millstone," which means, he's understood how the world works.

In the meantime, today as I wait for my patient,
I sit down near you,
to cool off
in the shade of your eyes.

37.

What about the survivors of rope, pistol, lethal drugs?
To understand them you have to talk to them, but how do you do that?
For them too you need a net, and years of patience.
They are still confused, or so fatuous they can't distinguish being alive from being dead.
They can't manage to tell their story, but why is that?
I am so stupid that it's taken me years to figure it out.
It's the trauma of falling that pulls those who jump, for a

time, out of their psychosis. They come out of their dreamlike state and are amazed, they don't recognize themselves in the suicide.
Another explanation: jumping is a sudden act, three seconds, often a relatively mild psychotic state is enough to push them and so it's easier to come out of.

I prefer the fallen.
They look out at the world from stunned and fearful eyes, as if it were the first time. They want to understand what has happened.
They want to talk to you. And they become attached to you. And to the treatment.

38.

You are extremely busy as you walk down the street, you must not be disturbed, you are occupied with something very serious. What is it?
Holding up your pants with two hands.

You go into a store, buy food, turn to the right, twist to the left, with two fingers you hold your pants, with the other three your bags. A true master.
I know, Giulio, your belt was taken away during your first mental health admission to prevent you from hanging yourself, but thirty years have passed since then! And for twenty years you've lived on your own in the city! And you manage a company!

I'm sorry. The past is the past.
This new life requires more self-respect.

39.

When it comes to death, perhaps more than fear,
it is the curiosity of finding out what's on the other side.
I will face death with the boldness of a busybody.

40.

When she arrived in front of me, the Lady stood still
and clearly pronounced:
you no longer have trains to miss,
you no longer have appointments to forget,
you no longer have outfits to get wrong,
you no longer have lovers to disappoint,
you no longer have bad impressions to avoid making,
you no longer have tears to swallow

now you are what you were at the beginning, before you were born,
an empty container to be returned.
And this container belongs to me.
I have come to take it back.

41.

Two deaths already tonight, and there are still three hours until dawn.
Heart attacks in terminal patients.
I am here on the medical ward for a consultation, I am about to leave and I briefly turn around to look. It's not over yet.
A shout. Two nurses find each other in the corridor: another one! The one who shouted points to the room.

They go in. Mumbles of pity and a sweetly whispered comment.
Then they shuffle out, get sheets, go in again. A moan.
(Perhaps for the waxy body, yellow under the neon lights?)
Whispers, armchairs moving, something falling and hitting the floor.
(Are they cleaning him?)
A nurse crosses the corridor with two IV bottles, enters another room. Silence. She reappears, crosses the corridor again.
The rustling of sheets.
(The empty body is an obscene shell, are they covering it?)
Steps again, a joke, a shrill laugh.
Where shall we put it? With the others?
Blunt metallic blows, the pitter-patter of footsteps.
The bed with the body comes out of the door, a nurse is pushing it.
The other follows with some bags.
They follow the corridor to its end, a door is opened, they push the bed with the bags on top through it, they close it again.
The nurses now walk towards me grumbling, they are talking about their plans for tomorrow.
They go into the kitchen, a telephone rings, someone answers, the gurgling of the coffee pot,
nothing more.

42.

The hour of the wolf is from two until four in the morning.
At that time there is a strange suspension in the air,
it is the time when hospital patients die.
It is an empty time, uninhabited, does not belong to humans.
The latest of the night owls have already turned in, and the earliest risers are yet to wake.
Those on the night shift slow down, become estranged from

themselves, their consciousness lets down its guard. A fragile person would say strange presences circulate. Rustles, calls, gusts of wind.
Personally, I don't need such subtleties.
When I walk the hospital corridors by night,
I find Death showing her face.
At that time of night she doesn't slip along the walls, she makes her rounds with a confident step.
It is cramped with two of us in the elevator,
she looks ahead, I down, neither speaks.
She gets out first
and starts sniffing around the beds.
Doctors and nurses kick her, she moves a little then quickly gets back to it.
Death doesn't appear suddenly, she doesn't swoop down from above with a glinting sword,
she's a stray nuzzling at your feet,
if you don't shoo her away she'll bite you,
once she has smelled you, she won't leave you alone.

43.

When is the right time to die?
Later.

44.

How nice it is when every nurse gives their opinion
on how they would like to kill or see dead
the most hateful patient on the ward.
Shot, hung, stabbed,
poisoned, suffocated,

burned, quartered.
The atmosphere relaxes as the coffee bubbles over.
Impaled, electrocuted, crushed, fallen, drowned, boiled, devoured.
The coffee cups are placed on the tablecloth and the sugar is taken from its hiding place.
Raped, skinned, blown up, stoned, throat slit, torn apart, splattered.
When the coffee is drunk, the two teams of nurses say goodbye.
One stays and one goes.

Spat out.

45.

Giulia, the most difficult ideas to understand in life
are the ideas of You and I.
I have devoted fifty years to figuring out the difference between You and I
and I have thought about it for many hours every day.
Every interview I have done has been an attempt to distinguish between You and I.
Over the years, I have begun to understand.

Perhaps it would have been better not to understand.
I know now for certain that when I die, it is I who will die.
Quite satisfying.
If I hadn't understood, maybe it would have been You who died.

Chapter Eight
Binding people

1.

I go to the ER for someone I don't know.
He is lying immobile on the stretcher, turned to face the wall.
Excuse me, sir, I am a doctor, what's the matter?
In a rapid motion he turns and strikes me, hard,
a punch in the face.
Face and glasses smashed.

As you, Adriano, wave at the crazy people outside the window,
there's no need to worry. You're right, they're not dangerous at all.
Pain is a reminder.

2.

Marcello, making a diagnosis is also a matter of distance.
The euphorics, always in a hurry and dressed for summer in the middle of winter, can be identified from a distance of forty yards.
The drunks and the drug addicts, with their swerving gait, from thirty yards.
The schizophrenics, mannered movements and strange outfits, from twenty yards.
The depressives, ashen and immobile, from ten.

The neurotics, from five yards and closer, but some mask it very well and it drops down to two.
Some neurotics are sly and you need to look into their eyes to see it: one yard.
Others don't talk, they are confused and you need to be less than two feet away to sniff it out.
Any farther is useless.
Some anxious, hysteric, mentally disabled patients
get right under you, one foot.
The slackers and the ball-breakers breathe in your face.
Under eight inches, only my wife.

3.

War wounds on Ward 77?
Four broken ribs
plus a finger on one hand and a toe on one foot.
Scratches, grazes, and hematoma.
Insults, attacks, threats.
All this and not even a tin medal to show for it.

4.

In the city the mad, in their apartments, can do whatever they like:
shout, stamp their feet,
bang their heads against the walls,
hang themselves, shoot themselves, die,
and nobody intervenes.
It is the new tolerant society.
But if they throw something out of the window,
a chair, a bottle, pee, poop, a cat, immediately there are traffic wardens, police, firefighters, the forest service, the air force, and

the navy. And they call us urgently to respond to the extremely serious situation.

Mad people, do you want to be left alone?
Then don't throw anything out of the window.
Politicians, do you want to abolish mental asylums? Get rid of windows.

5.

When progress is made in Medicine nobody demonizes the old methods, nobody blames those who practiced them.
That's not how it is here.
In Psychiatry the present is cleansed, relegating the bad to the past.
And that's why I would like to talk about binding people.

6.

I went up, with a nurse and a police officer, to an attic in the old town because you were sitting with one leg in and one leg out, straddling the windowsill, shouting at the diving swallows.
The alleyway is still, mothers look up in curiosity, then pull their children away.
You speak excitedly in a made-up language,
high on God knows what.
This room is not too big nor too small, one should be able to move around just fine,
which is important
because, in a few seconds, I don't know what,
but in a few seconds something is going to happen.

There are two windows in the room. One of us in front of each,
I at the door we came through.
But there is another door, that opens onto the terrace,
I see basil poking out of pots and the yellow of lemons,
I can already see you running over the city's rooftops.
I move, as if it meant nothing, toward the terrace,
I arrive, I position myself,
I turn around, you lash out.

7.

When a way of working has saved my life and that of my patients, I have difficulty speaking ill of it.
And if I hear somebody sitting at a desk speaking ill of it, I defend it.

8.

You tell me, Luca, in an earnest tone, that the psychiatric patient must be accepted in toto,
he and his illness, as a particular expression of the human,
and therefore any form of restraint must be rejected.
Luca, this approach has value for those who, like you, work with people whose condition is chronic, unchangeable.

In Emergency Psychiatry, it is the person who is accepted in their entirety, not the disease.
Otherwise we would allow the mentally ill to cross the street at a red light without intervening.
We would let the depressed commit suicide in front of our eyes.
We would let the manic wander into the tunnels of trains.
We would let the hallucinating climb down the balcony railings.

We would let the delirious turn against their neighbors with weapons.
We would let the alcoholics and drug addicts unleash their primitive rage.

9.

Nobody will stop you at the end of the day to ask, Why did you treat me, doctor?
Why did you restrain me?
Why didn't you leave me free like I was?

Somebody may however ask, Why didn't you treat me?
Why did you leave me at the mercy of myself?

10.

Filippo, you are scared that in the dark
someone will come from outside and kill you.
Bulletproofing your door is no use,
barricading your bedroom window is no use,
shutting yourself away in a prison is no use.
Filippo, the assassin is locked in the cell with you.

11.

You tell me that you can calm down a distressed and confused patient with words and body language.
Luca, the distressed and confused patient, by definition, does not understand words or body language.
You insist that you have done it many times.

Those patients were not distressed and confused.

12.

At the end of the talking, the end of the smiles, when the patient has you up against the wall,
what method is the simplest, oldest, cheapest, most natural, and most human?
Touch, of course.

13.

At the beginning something happens that frightens or angers the patient,
the nurses ask, What do you want? What's wrong?
Most of the time a bit of attention is enough, and even the fieriest of souls cools down.
But if everything is happening in the patient's head,
there is nothing that can be done.

Phase one is the gorilla phase.
The patient starts talking in a loud voice,
gesticulating, puffing up his chest,
walking fast, moving from room to room without warning,
he starts hitting the door, slapping it, trying to open it,
punching the wall, pushing the other patients around and so on. He is making it clear that he is here, he is angry
and he has the power to cause chaos.
If the gorilla has the gift of speech, he moves quickly onto threats:
he'll destroy everything or he'll murder everyone or he'll kill himself

if one of his requests is not fulfilled,
immediate discharge or that he be given a certain drug, often a coffee, a cigarette, changing bed neighbors, making his one hundredth phone call to his mother.
We try to stay calm, and all the while we are thinking,
It had to happen to me,
one hour before the end of my shift!
Who is the imbecile that made him angry? Who lowered his tranquilizers?
The old nurses immediately understand:
if they are quiet, sighing, it means it will end badly,
if they counterattack, in an equally loud voice, telling him to stop being an idiot, it will end well.

Phase two is the negotiations.
Would you like a coffee, cigarettes, phone calls, to change beds?
Here it comes, straight away.
Thank you, now I want to be discharged, immediately!
The nurses stall, we need to wait for your doctor, perhaps tomorrow,
see, we care about you,
if it were up to us we'd have satisfied your requests already, it's just that we'll get fired.
At this point we witness the miracle of patients who just an hour earlier seemed out of it, transformed into seasoned lawyers
responding blow by blow, vehemently claiming that we are beating around the bush.
Some nurses are great negotiators, UN worthy, so good they could be diplomats. When one of them is in, I make myself comfortable and watch and learn.
If words fail to produce the desired effect, it is time for "why don't you take some medicine?"
Something "very light" for your headache, constipation,
just vitamins

and in the meantime a double dose injection is prepared.
The patients can always smell the deceit and resist with indignation, demonstrating their contempt,
only few accept this honorable way out,
avoiding the final show of strength.
In this phase, while one nurse negotiates, the other sets to preparing the clamps and bandages.

Now it is our turn to be the gorilla and beat our fists on our chests.
We show the patient our strength,
how many of us there are, how united, how young and strong.
This is the crucial moment, just a few seconds determine everything.
The patient understands that he will not have another chance.
Either he accepts the bright orange triple injection
or he'll be bound.

Phase three is the restraint.
There have been countless guidelines written on restraint.
Writing or reading the guidelines is one thing,
being there on the day is another,
with a bad back, an unkind colleague,
bandages nowhere to be found
—they have always been borrowed, or broken—
another patient getting in the way, protesting relatives, a lost key, calls from the ER, a slippery floor, and the patient we plan to restrain all of a sudden brandishing a chair.
Fate throws the guidelines to the wind and puts us to the test.
The door is closed and we begin.
The only ones who can save us now are the patients themselves.

The schizophrenics don't want to do any harm, often they have a deep bond with us,
if we move with sureness they put up little resistance to the restraint, often they burst into tears,

life has pummeled them too much already to take another beating today.
The euphorics can do harm by accident, but not maliciously, they often apologize as they continue to hit you.
They smile as they hit.
But not all the patients are kind.
The addicts and the drunks don't have control and have no qualms about hitting you,
they're not thinking about the reprisal, which is what puts the brakes on the instinctive joy of doing harm in those with personality disorders.
The hysterics, with the excuse that they are ill and don't know what they're doing, can be nasty
and target the body with sophisticated malice.
The paranoid, afraid of being destroyed, fight tooth and nail in the final combat.
Even if experience has taught us to expect nothing more of larger patients, we continue to fear them and take a beating from the small ones.

Finally, having bound the patient to the bed, with great relief and in mystical procession,
we proceed to carry out the magic violet-colored injection, demanding everybody's attention as it is brought to the bed like a relic from the past.
It pacifies us all.

The fourth and final phase, is sharing memories around the campfire.
The patient sleeps and the nurses gather in the kitchen, checking one another over for wounds, scratches, and bruises.
They speak ill of absent colleagues, cowards, doctors, administrators, and work in general.
Then they reconstruct the events

benevolently insulting the patient,
and all his relatives to the sixth degree,
the brave and the courageous are thanked and the oafs are affectionately criticized.
The atmosphere relaxes, becomes warmer and lighter. Like tribal hunters in the firelight, memories from the past resurface: the toughest restraints, the acts of greatest heroism, the most painful wounds, the scariest moments and how they wriggled out of them, the funniest scenes,
that time Irma was restrained by a patient,
that time Giusi did the whole thing by herself,
former nurses are honored, those who with just a look, a word, a hand, could calm the most riotous.
And slowly the madness and violence is washed away.

14.

If a shower was sufficient to wash away the madness and violence that coats your skin as you work,
I'd shower ten times a day.

15.

To bind or not to bind is not the decision of a single psychiatrist, but of the management of the ward,
it is the ward who chooses to bind or not to bind, not the single doctor.

16.

The person who binds isn't evil, binding is hard work.

Evil is the person who abandons his patient.

17.

Yesterday on Ward 77, Francesco, the euphoric patient, the young one, decided to play tennis in the corridor,
imaginary tennis.
He didn't have a racket or a ball, but his movements were those of a tennis player; he is big and tall, running back and forth, and the corridor is narrow,
so if somebody tried to pass they would be crushed.
He refused his treatment in the afternoon. Bad sign.
After an hour we say to him, The tennis court is closing.
He says, No, it's my private court.
We tell him it's getting dark.
Then turn on the floodlights, I'll pay.
This leaves us in a bind. Francesco will play for hours. We insist on a sedative,
and he says, Can't you see I'm playing?
We confront him again as a trio, and he continues. It's the Italian Open.

With a manic, the first task is to catch him. He moves continuously, and if you manage to grasp him he slips through your fingers.
On top of that you need to be determined, decisive, and a bit unkind. How can you do that if the manic is making you laugh?
He laughs, you laugh. You fall into despair.
How can you even imagine being able to bind him? Manics get away by being nice.
Until one of us bursts out, Enough! Guys, do we want to do this or not? And we try.
Mania is an optimistic view of the world,

deceit is an option but not anger or the pleasure of doing evil.
The manic does not hit you on purpose,
however, especially if he is robust, he can do you a lot of harm because he bumps into you, gives you a slap, slips a finger into your eye, it's like dealing with a small child, but one who's bigger than you.
And indeed, after jumping to reach the ball, Francesco landed on Lino's foot.
Broken middle toe.

18.

How do you inject someone who is so distressed, Luca?
You need to hold them down whichever way possible.
If you do not want to use force, you must call public force, but what do you do while you're waiting? Let the patient run around freely for twenty minutes? A lot can happen in twenty minutes.

The police arrive, they hold the patient down and you give him an intramuscular injection.
It's not like in the movies where the guy immediately collapses, it takes at least a quarter of an hour, often one injection isn't enough.
After half an hour you have to do it all again, the police don't hang around.
Only an intravenous anesthetic takes immediate effect, but for that you need to call the anesthetist.
What's better, I wonder, being tied to the bed or a drug-induced coma?

I, by tying the patient to the bed, have everything secured in five minutes

and can use low doses of drugs with substantially fewer risks.
The patient remains conscious and I can talk to him, reassure him and ask him for information.
But each psychiatrist does what they know and what they can.
Faced with a distressed and confused patient, all roads are rocky.

19.

I go onto Ward 77 and ask for Ferdinando, they tell me he's been injured, and he's not the only one.
Massimo is also injured. Two of the toughest nurses!
Who hurt them? A woman? What bed is she in?
Tied to the bed I find a small, young woman, skin and bones, ninety pounds. I don't believe it. I go back,
That little sparrow injured both Ferdinando and Massimo?
They recount one of the most dramatic restraints of recent years,
the two of them were sure they could do it, but the little sparrow was a fury, she ambushed the nurses.
She wriggled, she thrashed, she bit, she scratched, she kicked, she spat.
A wild cat knocked two lion tamers out of action.

20.

If a nurse has a reputation for being strong and mean, they need only to make half of the effort to keep a patient calm.
Ferdinando, your reputation is so good, you need only to make a tenth of the effort.

21.

I have talked to colleagues who work in a zero-restraint department. They say that they avoid restraints by spending a lot of time talking to try to bring the patient around.

I am of the old school, I can't stand these infinite attempts at persuasion,
I find it much more violent and wild than a quick, strong, clean restraint.
Often, after the restraint, the mind clears and the insanity dissipates,
The rain eases and the sun comes out,
and when you go back into work the next day,
the patient smiles at you and says hello.
After hours of futile persuasion, however,
the insanity only overflows,
moves from the patient to you, fills the rooms,
permeates the walls, sticks to the ceilings,
blocks the air outlets, soaks into the floors.
You can no longer breathe.
You need to go home, but the madness doesn't leave you, it follows attached to your coat like a mangy dog.
When you come back to work you are tired and confused, and you find the patient tired and confused.

It takes two minutes to know whether a patient is persuadable or not,
and if they are not persuadable, why go on swimming upstream for hours in the madness?
But this is only my opinion, and I come from a school of restraint, I may be wrong.

22.

There is a hysterical patient, Luisa, who gets jealous whenever we strap someone to the bed.
Then she goes to the very end of the ward and starts screaming and breaking everything.

23.

Alfredo, the fact that yesterday I asked you the name of an antibiotic for a sore throat
does not authorize you to tell me about your father and your mother, from cradle to grave,
including how they met, the war, their escape from prison,
the bombardments, the hunger, the partisan struggle and your difficult birth
and to ask me, finally, if that's why you are anxious and can't sleep at night.
Alfredo, you are an internist, in twenty seconds you can give me the name of an antibiotic.
I, in twenty seconds, cannot give you psychotherapy.

24.

This morning, entering Ward 77, I managed less than a yard before I was stopped by a wall of solid, impenetrable stench.
In the distance I caught a glimpse of nurses in long green overshirts and masks and caps covering their hair, coming and going gesticulating,
a homeless man admitted in the night has taken his shoes off for the first time in a year.

Every minute, a worker takes their turn to come out of the ward to breathe.
The power of feet, stronger than fire, an earthquake, a blackout.
Forget meetings, ultrasounds, CAT scans, MRIs, transplants, moon landings. Wash his feet!
A tremendous operation, dark, dangerous, extremely complex, interminable.
Credit to the heroic workers.

25.

Today I decided not to restrain a patient.
I don't have scratches, I haven't sweated and I'm going home on time.
But I am not happy, like when you could have helped someone and you didn't.
He was delirious and refusing treatment. A robust guy, a tricky customer.

You can always find an excuse for not restraining a patient:
there are too few of us and we'll get hurt;
the team on the next shift will deal with it;
what do you think, if we force him to take the drugs tonight, will he get better?
if we bind him, we'll wake up the other patients;
if we bind him, we'll put our therapeutic alliance on the line;
his father is a lawyer, if we leave a scratch he'll press charges;
what harm is he doing being delirious?
his parents have always said yes to him, why should it be us to start saying no, tonight?
give him a depot! It'll last a month, and we can forget about it!

Every excuse is a good one and I don't remember which one we chose.
But I am sure that, thanks to our decision,
some time in the future,
someone will find themselves in a tricky situation.
Their problem.

26.

When I meet strangers at a party I conceal my job.
As soon as you let on that you're a psychiatrist, someone pops up who wants to teach you what Psychiatry is.
Electroshock is harmful, and what the sick people really need is understanding and music therapy,
antidepressants don't help, it is better to be treated with herbs or by taking a vacation.
I, when I meet a nuclear engineer, do not set out to explain to him how an atom or neutrino works,
nor how to manage a nuclear power plant.

27.

Certain patients are so lonely
that, to get you to lay your hands on them,
they break everything.

28.

Do you remember, Emilio, when everything between you and us was one big full-contact battle?

And now here we are addressing each other politely like English spinsters.
We talk with puckered lips,
but nobody is listening and everybody is thinking about their own business.
Do you remember when we used to push each other, pull each other's hair, scratch each other, and you would bite?
You had beautiful teeth, but how it hurt.

My best memories from childhood are the brawls between me and my brother.
Who do I play with now?
What do I go to work for? To talk?

29.

Fabia, you have been a nurse for many years,
And in order to be able to keep working in Psychiatry
you have lost all humanity,
but if you have lost all humanity, Fabia,
you cannot keep working in Psychiatry.

30.

I go to a seminar on restraint,
there is a colleague there who teaches how to do it.
He says in passing how many restraints he has done in his life,
it is the same number as I do in a year.
I went outside to take a walk in the park.

Why do we do so many restraints on Ward 77?
Are we evil? I do not feel evil.

Are we incapable? I do not feel incapable.
What is the trick? What is the mystery?

31.

The simplest method for not binding anyone,
is to not admit patients who need binding.
If we do not admit patients with alcoholism, personality disorders, drug addictions, organic psychosyndrome, dementia, those who are drunk or generally violent, who is left to be bound to the bed? The nurses themselves.
All you need to do to transform Psychiatry into Psychology
is refuse anyone who is distressed and confused.
The distressed patients will be bound by someone else.

32.

After many years of experience I can say
that the only real problem with binding someone to the bed
is knowing how to do it properly.
If you don't know how to do it properly, it's better to avoid doing it.

33.

The idea that it's possible to never restrain
is the presumption that reason and the heart can understand and placate all.
This presumption only increases the patient's anger.

Reason is the fly slipping down the wet glass. Let's allow man his anger.

34.

Marcello, look at the nurses sitting in the kitchen, they look as though they're doing nothing.
It's not true, they are listening.
You need experience and knowledge to listen to the sounds that come from the ward.
Listen in.
Neon lights, everything still. What do you hear?
Chatting between patients, footsteps, the opening of a cupboard door,
a chair moving, a moan,
a word shouted over and over again senselessly. Now a scream.
The nurses don't bat an eyelid.
Try asking, Who is that screaming? Alberto, they respond, he is fighting with Filippo.
At a certain point they get up, synchronized, you have not heard anything. What has happened? There was a quiet thud.
Pina has fallen and banged her head.
Just like parents with small children playing in the neighboring room, they listen
and they go and check, not when there's noise, but when there's silence.

35.

We might as well be clear.
When a person is restrained there are four roles, which are portioned out with a few nods and glances as we make our way over to the patient.

The immobilizer. That's the one who gets the patient in a neck hold and immobilizes the head, one arm, and chest.

He regulates the strength of the hold according to the reaction.
Hysterics and people with personality disorders understand the game
and collaborate from the first moment.
Manics, schizophrenics, and drunks do not understand and it is all much more difficult.
The immobilizer, if he is good, can drag the patient to the bed by himself.

The weight. That's the one who places himself on top of the patient on the bed and blocks the other arm, pelvis, and legs.
If he is good, he can do it alone.

The free-mover. That's the one who runs quickly around the bed and straps the four limbs.
If he is good, he can do it alone.

Then there's my role. I participate in all the restraints. I am not needed.
I can do it alone.

36.

When you tell me something, you start with the background from three days earlier.
You describe in detail what you ate, who you met, how you slept.
I ask you to get to the point, it's coming now, you say. And it doesn't come. Is this the problem? No, it's coming now.
Enough, I get up to dismiss you. You burst into tears as if I am about to cut your throat.
I give up.

I sit back down but I set off hunting bears in Canada, along a river where fish are jumping.
You continue describing minutiae and setbacks,
until finally you get to the point, the big reveal
and you stop with your hands to the sky and look at me, to see the effect.
But now I am in Canada.
You await my comments.
I, who have heard nothing, assume an air of painful joint participation, eyes lowered, shoulders narrow, as if at a funeral.
You scrutinize me attentively for a few seconds, then,
Doctor, no one understands me like you do!

37.

I come back from the Emergency Room with a girl strapped to the stretcher,
Giulia sees her, her eyes turn glassy and she protests, Restraint is a violent act,
it takes away freedom, it needs to be banned.

Giulia, you are right.
But violence and freedom are matters of psychology, not psychiatry.
The severe psychiatric patient has no awareness of the meaning of violence and freedom.
For him the matter of existing or not existing is more relevant.
Often he needs to be restrained in order to pull himself back together as a whole, to have a sense of himself, to live.
If you give him kindness and freedom, you kill him.

You look at me with doubt, you try to understand but remain unconvinced.

Psychologists, unbelievably, live in a psychological world!

38.

A forty-year-old man brings his sixteen-year-old son into the ER and says, You need to admit him, he's mad.
I talk to the son, It's me who brought my dad here, he's crazy, you have to admit him.
These games of *guess who's the mad one* keep you in the ER for hours, and in the end you have gone mad!

39.

If you were to ask me for an image that's symbolic of Emergency Psychiatry
it is binding,
reuniting shattered fragments,
pulling together mind and body, reunifying the person,
like a cast resets bones.
Make, from pieces, a whole.

40.

We come into the world
not when we leave our mother's body,
but when our mother embraces us and recognizes us
and, without words, contains us still within her,
within this matrix is where we build ourselves.

The sacredness of this primitive embrace
flickers and reverberates

in some of our restraints.

41.

The art of binding people.
Binding people to the bed.
Binding people to you.
Binding people to reality.
Binding people to themselves.
Binding people is an art.
Unknowable.

42.

Marcello, this is easy. If a patient holds a hand on their upper chest, they are anxious.
Hand to the left over the heart: hypochondriac.
Hand on the lower chest: depressed.
Hand on the abdomen: depressed but less aware of it.
Hand on the groin: hysteric.
If, however the hand is on the head or the legs, don't even try: you'll need a real specialist for that.

43.

If you want to know the soul of a psychiatrist,
look at which patients they treat.
Tito treats only hysterics.
Edoardo only bipolars.
I only schizoids
and Rufo only rich fakers.

44.

I thought that this job would bring with it a line of young women in love,
but instead I am followed by a line of old women
all angry.

45.

I have spent two hours vacantly ruminating on life's big questions.
When you get home, Anna, you slap me round the head
and ask, Did you buy bread?
Bread? As I get up and run to the bakery,
I think of my friend Elia who sailed all the way to India
in search of the zen master. Do not think, do.
My zen master is right here, clattering around in the kitchen.

46.

It was not just compassion that brought about the closure of mental asylums, but drugs.
Sixty years ago people had to be bound to the bed for weeks, until the crisis was placated. Today the distressed person is bound for the time it takes for the drugs to kick in.
It can be hours or days. From delirium tremens to hysteria, there is an order in the chaos, and we always respect the time it takes. Bets are placed.
Acute psychosis, which is magmatic and immeasurable like nothing else in nature, travels with a stopwatch in hand.
Always on time.

47.

I want to tell the truth: in the past I have restrained many people, which I have ceased doing, but not yet regretted.

Chapter Nine
Words are straw

1.

Adriano, when I, a young and eager doctor,
turn up at the Mental Health Center ready to learn
you tell me, There's nothing to learn.
What about mental illnesses? They do not exist.
So where do I start? It's all over.
But I've just arrived. And you can leave again.
Is there nothing I need to do? We've already done everything.
My generation has settled the score with madness.

2.

I won't trouble anyone. I'll breathe quietly.
After you, Previous Generation, only post people are born,
post-closing of mental asylums[1].
For years they have said to me, What do you think you know,
you who are post?
And there I was thinking I was normal.

[1] The Italian Law 180, "The Reform of Psychiatric Care," also known as the Basaglia Law, was approved in 1978 and ushered in the closing down of psychiatric hospitals, replacing them, in part, with community-based services. The most fervent supporters of the law considered it sufficient to eliminate mental illness.

3.

Adriano, how can your generation have settled the score with madness,
if every newborn has to elbow their way through the madness?
If every newborn has to fight to stick their head out of the sludge of madness?
If every newborn, in order to breathe,
has to shake off the thousand hands of madness?
Adriano, humanity wasn't extinguished with your generation.

4.

Giulia, you tell me that my white coat is filthy and that I should change it.
Let me see: this one's a bloodstain,
this is a spit stain, this is ink, this is sweat
and this is where Franco kicked me.
In that moment Rufo walks past in an immaculate coat,
brilliant white,
as if he has an ironing lady following him everywhere.
You look at him admiringly. That's a real doctor.

5.

Adriano, telling a psychiatric patient
that mental illness does not exist
is like telling the patient that his experience does not exist,
that he does not exist.

6.

I do not know any psychiatrists who died in the war for psychiatric reform,
nor do I know any martyrs or invalids from the battle for Law 180.
I do not know of doctors who risked their lives
fighting at the walls of the mental asylums,
I know of doors that were opened by the struggles of the people, of trade unions and of politics, I know of doctors who became head physicians well before they were forty, to whom it was said, Enter and take.
They gave you a province to govern that had already been conquered.

Do not now demand a horse-mounted monument.

7.

To prescribe medicines and then leave
is like handing out horoscope cards,
like setting a message in a bottle on the sea.
Depressed people suffer from guilt, theirs is a moral problem,
they do not understand what the medicines are for.
Manics are fine as they are and do not want medicines that will depress them.
Schizophrenics are attached to their voices and don't even know who you are.
Paranoid people are convinced that you want to poison them.
Those with personality disorders swallow the whole bottle that same evening.
The neurotics are the only ones who read the label and slavishly follow it, up until the first side effect,

then they decide not to take them.
Marcello, you are not the kind of intern who says, Take these medicines, and sees the job as done.
That moment is when your work begins.

8.

In the Mental Health Center there is a private lounge with some old armchairs and brown curtains.
The room where I see my patients opens onto this room.
Summer, winter, spring, and fall,
before every appointment, I open a door and find the same colleagues sitting on the armchairs.
Morning, afternoon, and night.
Monday, Tuesday, Wednesday, Thursday, Friday, and Saturday.
Sometimes they bring something from the café to sip on,
or to stir with their long spoons, and they lick their fingers,
sometimes they ask one another questions from a magazine psychology quiz and laugh and cackle as if they are at the hairdresser,
sometimes they look pensive as if waiting at the gate in an airport, then suddenly get agitated as if outside a delivery room,
other times they watch out of the window as if awaiting a ship,
they feverishly discuss who is the most beautiful
who in the department gets the most sex
and they ask my opinion
as I see a patient out or invite one in,
other times they exchange recipes or phone numbers of plumbers with the head physician.
The patients, when they come into my room, ask me quietly,
Who are those people outside?
I don't know the answer.

9.

Edoardo, do you remember when we used to work at the Mental Health Center?
You would make a home visit to a schizophrenic patient and find yourself being
an electrician, marriage counselor, family doctor, cook, interior designer,
personal trainer, plumber, administrator, gardener, vet, brick-layer,
tailor, ironer, cobbler, mailman, TV repairman,
janitor, taste-tester, cleaner, tea master,
hairdresser, stockman, coalman, chiropodist,
bouncer, catcher of dogs, mice, cockroaches.

Do you remember, Edoardo?
What fun we had.
Then we transferred to the hospital, and we had to be psychiatrists.

10.

I have spent my life trying to convince thousands of people of the fact that they are ill
and it would be good for them to get better.
Other colleagues have spent their lives trying to convince illustrious audiences of the fact that mental illnesses do not exist.
Do we have the same job?

11.

Do you remember, Edoardo, when the nurses were in charge?

I would often visit patients alongside Thea. Every sentence I said to the patient, she would intervene with, No, that's not how it is! And she'd say the exact opposite.
The patient went home reassured.

As I spoke, she would silently express her dissent with a face of disgust.
One day I carelessly told her to be quiet, and she locked herself in silence for weeks
and when I asked for her opinion, she said,
If you want to be in charge, go ahead, but I will not tell you what I think.
Just like my wife.

12.

Psychiatry is one big game of snakes and ladders.
You take Mario and move him from the day center to the hospital.
Then you move him into the Therapeutic Community.
Then you move him into secure accommodation.
Then you move him into the day center.
Then you slide back to the beginning.
The hope is that on one of these journeys Mario disappears.
But the magic trick does not quite work, and the rabbit does not go back into the hat.

13.

Depots are the future. We'll see our patients once a month, five minutes, ciao.
No more physical contact.

No more arguing.

14.

Marcello, in Psychiatry words are powerless.

For the confused and mentally ill, words are nothing but sounds,
echoes, of echoes, of echoes,
reflections, of reflections, of reflections,
a dream, of a dream, of a dream.
For schizophrenics words mean everything and nothing,
they mean a thing and its opposite.
For the depressed words are a sentence.
For euphorics they are just a game.
For those with personality disorders, a threat.
For neurotics they are a sharpened blade.

Words are not a light that drives away ghosts in the night
nor firewood to keep dry for the cold winter,
nor food to store in the pantry,
nor a comforting lullaby.

Words are straw.

15.

Still devoted to that age-old mission of patrolling
the doorways and gardens in the hunt for cigarette ends,
the index and middle fingers of your right hand yellowed by nicotine,
you bend over, pick up a stub with a trembling hand,
check it over with a discerning gaze, holding it up in the air

then you examine the horizon to see who is coming and going,
who is smoking or not,
who might give you some change.

Seeing you here, bent over on the wide driveway of the ex-asylum, reminds me how much we used to smoke at the Mental Health Center.
One meeting in the morning and one in the afternoon, for years.
Twenty of us enclosed in a room and at least ten cigarettes each, two hundred cigarettes. Square feet of smoke.

And the topics of discussion. Whether to wear a white coat or not, whether to address the patient formally or not,
whether mental illnesses were caused by the parents, the teachers, the principals,
whether doctors and nurses were equal or whether the doctors should obey,
whether the pharmaceutical industry was financing Psychiatry, and how to resist it.

I never understood the last topic.
I was and am still convinced
that Psychiatry is financed by the cigarette factories.

16.

Chefs can identify a dish with their eyes closed, from the smell.
Marcello, would you be able to make a diagnosis using only your nose?

The depressed smell of damp laundry left to dry indoors, of herbal tea, mothballs, musk, menthol,

of sheets piled up for years, or old blankets on ancient sofas.
If they remove their shoes you smell nothing.

The euphorics smell principally of sweat,
they stink of petrol, the street, of spices.
Best to keep a distance from their socks and underwear.

The schizophrenics smell of their little vices: cigarettes, coffee, alcohol,
the most severe of dried filth, feces, and urine.
It is a dense, mottled odor.

Those with personality disorders smell of hashish, cigarettes, glue.
Cheap aftershave.

The homeless smell of wet cardboard,
of mold, dust, putrid, necrotic.
It is a sour odor, intense.
If they take off their shoes, there's nothing for it.

The neurotics emit delicate fragrances.
Painstakingly selected perfumes, of which I do not know the names. Lavender, gentian, various flowers.
If they take off their shoes, it is a pleasure to be around.

You, Marcello, smell of aftershave, I of swimming pool, and Giulia's skin makes heads turn.

17.

Giulia, the important thing in this job
is not what you say or do
but being there.

If you are there, the patient will do everything by themselves.

18.

Giulia, don't plant your words in dry land,
in the wrong season
or when the field is covered in crows.
Store your words away for when the land is humid,
the season opportune and the crows faraway.

19.

Rufo, you have the problem of struggling to find just the right phrase for the Boston conference. I have the problem of treating Filippo every week for ten years.
Rufo, if you deliver your just-right phrase in Boston, everyone will applaud. If I say the same phrase to Filippo, he will eat my tongue, hand, and arm.
Do not bring me a just-right phrase back from Boston, bring me a gun.

20.

It takes a dirty language, full of holes, a whorelike, cantankerous language, a shaky and cruel language, or even an intellectual, snobbish, scornful language.
It takes crooked words, assassin words, words of sprites who seize realities that do not exist,
kaleidoscopic words that contain mutating realities,
forklike words that will pierce infinitesimal realities,
ambiguous words that each interprets as they like.

This is why I mumble, break words in half,
interrupt conversations, sit in silence.
To make myself better understood.

21.

Anna, inside me there is the echo of the tragedy of the world.
Paolo, take out the trash
or I will make you hear the echo of the tragedy of the world.

22.

Poetic is the hurt of love, regret, grief,
poetic is the tragic pain that finds reason, revenge, release,
unpoetic is this pain, monotonous, slow, insatiable, abducting.
Poetic is nostalgia, unpoetic is depression.
Poetic is imagination, unpoetic is delirium.
Poetic is fear, unpoetic is angst.
Poetic is desire, unpoetic is dependence.
Poetry stops at the door of Psychiatry.

Where the spade of poetry does not enter, the earth is hard, dry,
infertile, and cold.
We work with unpoetic pain.

23.

Words are used at psychiatric conferences,
but a problem that can be defined with words
is not a psychiatric problem.

24.

Giulia, you ask me whether you should address patients formally or informally.
The depressives nod, groan, and if they speak they address you formally.
Speaking formally to a depressed person is a mark of respect.
The euphorics are enthusiastically informal, we are all brothers in this great world.
Speaking formally to a euphoric is a precaution.
The schizophrenics are confused by both the formal and the informal.
Speaking formally to a schizophrenic patient is best.
Those with personality disorders and drug addicts choose a conspiratorial informality: you understand me, we are all wretched and delinquent.
Speaking formally to someone with a personality disorder is a protection.
The hysterics skip the informal, and where possible move straight to the physical.
Speaking formally to a hysteric is an act of prudence.
The neurotics, if an informal phrase slips out, are shocked,
lower their heads, turn red and never come back,
for them speaking informally is a sexual proposition.

I know that I should speak formally to everybody,
and I try, I swear I try, but I don't manage,
and clumsily garble a mixture of the two.

25.

Why is it that someone who has experienced a stomachache
does not consider himself a surgeon,

yet someone who has experienced anxiety or depression considers himself a psychiatrist?

26.

I am like the lizards on the walls. If you try to catch them, they'll leave their tail in your hand as they escape.
These days I am without my tail, Sara, and I blame you.

27.

Another gathering to discuss psychoanalysis. Lawyers, engineers, teachers. I do not understand what they are talking about. When they invite me to give my opinion, I look like an idiot.
I hate psychoanalysis.

Sirs, madams, I say clearly, I know nothing about the interpretation of dreams. That is not my job.
My patients do not talk about their nocturnal dreams, they live inside of them.
I do not look for interpretations, I look for a rope to pull them out.

28.

To deny the existence of madness by saying that we are all equal is to invalidate the diversity of the other, painting everything gray.
In the era of asylums the mad were excluded from the city, today they are excluded from the mind. Total stigmatization.
A culture that attempts to talk of the human

but that ignores psychiatry,
is blind and incomplete.
We do not need to say that we are all equal, we need to recognize our differences.

29.

Leaving the hospital I place my feet on the ground.
It is still solid.
I make dinner. Before going to sleep, one more look out of the window.
The sea is a sheet of shimmering steel.
The stars and the moon are each in their place.
Fireflies float around.
Leaves lightly rustle.
Somewhere a frog croaks.
I close the window and go to bed.

Chapter Ten
Tortula muralis

1.

I am still dragging my pile of bones around the old buildings of Genoa.
Soon I will take my leave and these buildings will remain unchanged, just as they were the first time I saw them.
Generations change, the scenery stays the same.
I thank, on the threshold, the scenographer, the other leads, the extras, and the fine audience,
a special round of applause for the light technician,
everybody has had marvelous and clear ideas.
As for the writer, I have no idea where he's going with this.

2.

Gino, American movies teach us to never quit.
Gino, who can teach me to give me up?
Since I've been getting older, giving things up is dry bread,
the salt of every day, my barefoot companion,
it is the pain that doesn't go away, the drizzle,
a stride that does not lengthen, a breath that has become short,
it is the dish of the day on the menu, the date in the diary, the note on the dresser,
it is every day's good morning and good night.

3.

Signor Alfredo, starting treatment with a psychotic person is like starting a journey over land and sea to the edges of the world.
I am too old, my feet are unsteady. I get out of breath on mountain trails. I suffer with the humidity.
I'd be a burden, not a guide.
I'm not going away anymore.
Signor Alfredo, for your son I recommend a younger colleague.
His name is Marcello.

4.

Marcello, today as always we walk past the Oncology unit, look at that small crowd of patients, renewing itself by the day. Their eyes, the look of expectation.
Why do they hardly ever call us here?
Because the evil that we fight is not pain, not fear, not vacillating hope.
It is not the loss of life,
but the loss of self.

He who cries knows who he is.
We stop only for the one who is blind with bewilderment in his eyes.
It is beside him that we sit down.

5.

If it is true that we soothe the pain of others because we have pain inside of us,
how big must my pain be?

6.

Today on Ward 77 it feels like the day after a nuclear explosion. Marcello and I are trudging around inside heavy protective anti-radiation suits, we look and talk through a fogged-up glass and we wear thick gloves.
Around us are vaporized lives,
disintegrated lives,
lives printed on the wall.

7.

When you meet a new patient, the question to ask yourself is, Are they living before, during, or after the end of the world? They are completely different situations.
If it is during, you see buildings, the city, time collapsing around you.
But a catastrophe is always on the horizon. Even if years, decades have passed, you still feel the echo of the big bang.
Few patients live in other days.
Few live in the cool morning or the serene evening of a tranquil day of light rain
and come to you carefree, just for a chat.

8.

Adriano, you who say that madness does not exist,
tell me what is this pain that I feel in my chest,
that runs through me like a river in spate,
and pulls in trees and houses,
and has no source, and has no mouth,
and has no name, and has no substance

and proceeds from nothing toward nothing
and makes of me its floor, its bottom, its bed.

And reassuring would be the end of the world, if only it were true,
and reassuring would be death, if only it were true,
and to be able to know again, in dying, who it is who is dying.

9.

Do not bring me maps, satellite photos, railway timetables of the city you once were,
do not bring me planning regulations, development projects, municipality budgets.
Elena, tell me what you smelled when you woke up in the mornings, make me hear the sounds rising from the embankment, the colors of the buildings surrounding the gardens,
and if you looked for shade, what route you took to go into town, and if you sought the sun,
how rough were the surfaces of walls when you ran your hand along them, and the sounds of the bells and from where the sounds came, the near ones and the far,
was it hot or was it cold, and before falling asleep what was the last sound that you heard?
Elena, is there any other wood or stones with which to rebuild?

10.

One often comes out of a psychological crisis with a more mature view of themselves and the world.
From a psychiatric crisis nothing is gained. But sometimes it happens.

One who has come through a psychiatric crisis with particular

lucidity is oppressed for months by the fear that everything could collapse all over again:
their identity, their feelings, their ideas, the very atomic matter around them,
unforeseeably.
With time this distressing apprehension mellows
and in its place grows a consciousness of the fragility of everything,
these people acquire a sense of the ephemeral.
They are the closest people to reality.
They have respect and attention for themselves and for others,
they use words that mean something,
they tend to the essential, they are sensitive, frugal, sincere.
They do not steal your time, they always give you something.
It is wonderful to be near them.

Then over time they heal completely.
They forget everything
and become false once again.

11.

The best people are those who do not forget that they have died mentally
and been reborn.

Some of them make brilliant psychiatrists.

12.

Marcello, you must have a sense of your patients' hard core.
It's the part that holds back potential mental collapse,
it's where catastrophe stops,

it's our last frontier.

Knowing if it exists and how solid it is helps us to know how much the patient is risking, how much he can suffer
and the necessary extent of our caution.

The depressives and the euphorics come and go bouncing on a tall trampoline.
The schizophrenics live plunging endlessly, twirling and evolving as they go.
The borderlines you see drop like lead, and crash soon after.
Those with personality disorders are made of stone, hard and indestructible: they make you crumble.
The neurotics are always about to be swallowed, but are never swallowed, by quicksand.

I do not believe I have a hard core,
I live on an infinite sloping plane.

13.

Do not seek total awareness of existing.
Each person lives in a fog of varying density.
Choose your place on the slope, and build yourself a home.

14.

Giulia, meeting with a patient is not the imposition of reason over madness,
it is the meeting between two madnesses.
Just hope that yours is the more human and the more wise.

15.

Marzia, you are eternally in a nascent state.
You are on edge with excitement, you are always on the verge of doing something electrifying,
You adjust your hair, change your dress, find new shoes to run who knows where.
Always breathless, eyes always made-up, always in uncomfortable heels.
Marzia, you are always in a nascent state but nothing is ever born.

16.

Livio and I visit the home of a euphoric patient, the neighbors called us. She lives alone in a luxurious apartment in Carignano and opens the door to us in an evening dress.
We are in her baroque salon, mirrors ten feet high, a grand piano, and many pink armchairs.
Let me say goodbye to the piano, she says, she sits down and begins playing a Mozart sonata.
The music is nice, I am too embarrassed to interrupt her. How long does a Mozart sonata last?
From the door to the stairwell an old man with a violin enters, he sits down and begins accompanying her.
Now two little old women and a mother with a child arrive and sit down to listen.
Then a young couple, a man with a hat, and a manual laborer.
The concert swells through the building down to the front door, people from the street rush in too.
We will have to wait.
On the final note everyone comes to shake her hand, to thank her.
A little old woman whispers to us, Treat her well, young gentlemen, she's been a bit funny lately,

but she is so sweet when she is well.

17.

Giulia, our patients are not skeins for us to unravel,
they are sacks that have split and been patched up a thousand times.
What you have found is not the golden thread, the mark of the past,
it is just a blemish.

18.

Yesterday, Emilio, in your euphoric tour of the hospital, you ended up in the morgue,
and you started telling the relatives not to cry
and you began consoling the dead.
You were talking to them, moving their arms, and modifying their faces to make them smile.
The outcome: one black eye, one broken rib, and a loose golden tooth.
Emilio, laugh as much as you like, but stay away from the morgue.

19.

Chiara, when you are depressed you think that a good doctor should not waste his time treating a worthless person like you.
How can I treat you, Chiara, if when I take an interest in you, you think it means I am an incompetent doctor?

20.

Marcello, immersing yourself in psychosis is like going underwater, it is not easy,
the majority of people can't even swim.
Many are free divers, few are scuba divers, very few are deep-sea divers. Then there are the amphibians.

Look at Edoardo. He is sitting in among the mad, wearing only a T-shirt, beard long, hair uncombed,
he laughs and jokes with them, not talking
—they understand each other in ways we cannot conceive—
now he is reading and writing an article at their table, not bothered by the noise and commotion.
Now they are laying the table and he will eat with them.
If you did not know him, you'd take him for a patient.
It is not clear if he's happier with them or with us.
Edoardo is an amphibian, a frog.
Like frogs, he needs to live at the border between land and water,
and if he gets too far away he'll shrivel up and die.

21.

I never understood why the patients of Clara the psychologist,
when they leave her office, look so happy, so sure of themselves,
while my patients stare at the ground, sad and insecure.
Then I understood: Clara the psychologist finds the culprit.
Parents are the best culprits, but the following also work well:
siblings, cousins, grandparents, friends,
husband, boss, lover, the dog, midwife, kindergarten teacher, mother-in-law, the neighbors,
preschool mates, colleagues, the plumber, God, politicians, the weather.

Having found the culprit, all they need to do is rebel, push the patient toward disobedience, invective, subterfuge.
The patients are like teenagers at war,
if someone asks them the time, they respond,
How dare you talk to me! You ruined my life!
Having eliminated the culprit, an even more fun phase begins: discover what we most like to do and do it, without hesitation.
At this point patients are seen abandoning their wives and children to run away with their twenty-year-old lover, leaving secure jobs to open a bar in the Caribbean, throwing themselves into homosexual relationships, heading off on round-the-world trips on a sailing boat, signing up to meditation retreats in the Sardinian mountains.
And if that doesn't work, all they need to do is find another culprit, and off they go!

How nice it would be to have a culprit at hand for all my problems.
But if you are born a cat, is it by any chance the fault of your parents who are cats?
Being a cat is a tragedy, like so many other facts of life.

22.

Desire means nothing in the face of mood,
it is a weather vane blown by the wind.

23.

Reason only adorns with rational explanations
that which our mood has already decided.

24.

Every psychiatrist, with every single one of his patients, forms a separate universe,
a separate stellar system,
in which the same laws of physics apply,
but with different masses, velocities, orbits, gravitations, atmospheres. Everything is different.
Each time a psychiatrist commits to and becomes part of one of these unique universes, he is the best.
Marcello, you have just said a phrase to Alberto that you heard from me yesterday: I have made my Psychiatry,
you create yours.

25.

I have spent my life never far from the Beast.
I have never looked it in the eye, but it has always been there,
its stench, its breath, its shadow,
its rasping heart, the shift in the air when it moved. It was there.
I have never harmed it, nor captured it, nor tamed it, least of all finished it off and butchered it, like one should.
It has never bitten me, torn off or devoured a limb.
It has been there, I have been there. We have simply watched each other.
The meaning of my life.

26.

You can only manage to work in Psychiatry if you can have fun.
I had fun for years.
Not all the years:

not the first years—too many illusions,
not the last years—too much paperwork,
not the middle years—too much hard work.

In an infinite prison, I felt free.

27.

And after many years I find myself here again,
dealing with useless pain.
Pain that does not teach, does not regenerate, does not renew.
Not the pain of growth but of imprisonment.
Not the pain of pruning but of death.
Pain that does not end in healing, does not end in necrosis and amputation. Pain that does not end ever.
Be infinitely blessed, pain that is useful, be infinitely damned, pain that is useless.

28.

And after the words, what remains of us, Enrica?
A window left ajar,
two lopsided chairs,
a half-closed door.
At the bottom of the stairs a cough,
a look,
a greeting.
The outside door closing.
Alone again.

Returning to the room, I find your scent.
In the still rapt air I almost struggle to walk.

In the silence my footsteps are thuds and the closing of a drawer an explosion.
A gust of wind and everything slowly disintegrates.
The echo of our final words is extinguished, the sounds of the city float up.
A fly enters, dives under the table, bolts up high, encircles the lamp.
It's all over.

Something sweet lingers in my suspended soul,
it's not to do with the *what* and the *why*,
the words that you said, that I said.
It is to do with your solitude, Enrica, and mine.

And I think, my day is made up of so many small goodbyes.
That is my trick for getting to the evening:
make a habit of the thing I fear most.

29.

Tortula muralis, moss that makes the walls soft for our hands
—and the ants—
unchanged for four hundred million years.
You have not developed roots, trunks, flowers.
Nor feathers, tusks, an upright position.
You don't bother getting in line on the evolutionary scale to reach intelligence, self-consciousness, contemplation of God.

Tortula muralis, you will never understand anything of the universe.
Or, perhaps, the one who has already understood everything is you.

30.

Here I am running down the San Leonardo hill with clogs on my feet
trying to catch a patient who has escaped from the ward.

Escaping from Psychiatry is not impossible, you just need to crouch down behind the door and wait for Dr. Milone to return from an evening consultation.
When I open the door and enter, an idiotic smile plastered upon my face, you slip out behind me. If you're sneaky, I won't even notice.
People escape from Psychiatry and always will.
It isn't a big deal, it's part of the game, the therapeutic relationship. The patients enjoy it
and deep down we're happy too: one fewer.
But if the patient is an involuntary hospitalization, it's completely different. A serious ward would never let an involuntary hospitalization escape.

So here I am running after you, Piero, at three in the morning in the deserted center of Genoa, my white coat billowing behind me and clogs slapping clack! clack!
A ghost.
But isn't Genoa beautiful by night.

You run in pajamas and bare feet, you have an advantage,
you're lighter,
but I don't want to remove my clogs, the street is filthy with excrement and shards of glass.
Luckily your advantage is reduced by all the drugs I've given you, which I'm grateful for,
you're getting tired, you're running upwind.
I don't manage to reach you and you don't manage to lose me, but time is on my side,

I'm a cyclist, I'm used to resistance.
Sooner or later I'll catch you.

What austere beauty in the buildings, the shimmering lights, the peace, the silence,
Genoa reveals itself, opens its arms, if only I could stop . . .
But no, we run at breakneck speed—clack! clack! clack!

We pass the shutters of the best gelateria in the city and find each other again in Piazza De Ferrari. Not a soul to be seen, it's all ours.
You do a lap of the fountain, me behind. A group of drunks appears from the city center and, seeing us, they stop singing, there is a ghost chasing a sleepwalker.

I catch a glimpse of you launching yourself down Vico San Matteo, dropping precipitously down to the sea. Me behind.
Clack! clack! Piazza De Ferrari echoes at night. A policeman, on instinct, runs after us.
He's running in boots.
How beautiful the strip of stars above the alleys.

Piazza Caricamento. You're done,
if I don't catch you, you're headed for the sea.
You stop, wheezing, leaning against the railing. I reach you and stand beside you, also wheezing.
For a moment each of us thinks only of breathing, then I suggest, sighing, We could run away to Corsica, what do you say?

That's when the policeman arrives.

31.

And while two patients shout, a nurse curses, two come to blows, another complains, one is on the telephone sorting his own business, the radiators don't work, there are no pens, a colleague protests, Why have you admitted him if he's fine?
And the patient protests, Why have you admitted me if I'm fine?
I continue to wander around, spectacles on, in search of the pain of others.

32.

You, who are staying, be kind.
Tell me when Gina starts to talk.
Tell me when Emilio no longer laughs.
Tell me when Filippo no longer hears voices.
Tell me when Tommaso leaves his house.
Tell me when Lucrezia comes back from wherever it is she has wound up.
Just a smile and a nod of the head.
I'll know.

Author's Note

I started working in a Mental Health Center in 1980, a little after they were established. From 1988 to 2016 I worked on a psychiatric ward in a hospital. That is almost forty years of life and of Psychiatry, which this book accounts for in a completely personal manner, with no respect for chronology. The fragments that constitute these pages are mixed up, placed side-by-side for their assonance and their contrast, gathered by theme, embracing the entire duration of my professional life.

Many things have changed over the years: there are no longer kitchens on the wards, and nobody would ever dream of creating an interview room from a broom cupboard.

But above all the drugs and the guidelines have changed, and the use of restraint has been drastically reduced.

I am not one who is nostalgic for bygone Psychiatry: the question is not whether to restrain or not restrain, but whether to practice or not practice good Psychiatry. The true difference lies in not abandoning the patient.

The characters I have described here do not correspond to real individuals. I note that I nearly gave the terrible Rufo the name Fabio, my middle name: there is thus a game of mirrors even with the characters who seem farthest from myself, and with the patients too. I speak, playfully, of a few critical or ridiculous aspects in a bigger picture that is generally remarkably positive, peopled by hundreds of splendid colleagues with whom I have had, for years, the honor and pleasure of working.

*

Thank you to Giovanni Profumo, without whose stubbornness this book would not have found the light.